TEACHING HEALTH-CARE WORKERS

Related Macmillan titles
For teachers of health care workers

Health Care Today — *training exercises for health workers in community based programmes* M Johnston and S Rifkin (1987) *TALC*

Partners in Evaluation — *Evaluating development and community programmes with participants* M-T Feuerstein (1987) *TALC*

Teaching and Learning with Visual Aids — *Program for International Training in Health (INTRAH)* (1988) *TALC*

The Church Health Educator B Wecker and I H Stober (1989) *TALC*

Talking AIDS — *A guide for community work* G Gordon and T Klouda (1989) *Co-published with IPPF*

For health care workers

Where There is No Doctor — *A village health care manual* D Werner (International Edition 1979 Africa Edition 1987) *TALC*

A Community's Road to Health M A Tregoning and D Dominic (1989)

Better Child Care M A Tregoning and G C Bova (1985) *TALC*

Nutrition Manual for Community Workers in the Tropics — *Caribbean Food and Nutrition Institute* (1987) *TALC*

Happy Healthy Children — *A child care book* J Hampton (1985) *TALC*

Healthy Living, Healthy Loving J Hampton (1987) *TALC*

Healthy Mothers, Happy Babies J Hampton (1991) *TALC*

Know Your Body M Skeet (1986)

All About Drink and Drug Abuse A McCall Smith (1990)

General tropical community health titles

My Name is Today — *An illustrated discussion of child health, society and poverty in less developed countries* D Morley and H Lovel (1986) *TALC*

The Struggle for Health — *Medicine and the politics of underdevelopment* D Sanders (1985) *TALC*

How to Measure and Evaluate Community Health J McCusker (1983)

District Health Care — *Challenges for planning, organisation and evaluation in developing countries* R Amonoo-Lartson, G J Ebrahim, H Lovel, J Ranken (1984) *ELBS*

Community Diagnosis and Health Action F J Bennett (1980)

Primary Health Care — *reorienting organisational support* G J Ebrahim and J P Ranken (eds) (1988) *TALC*

Social and Community Paediatrics — *Caring for the rural and urban poor* G J Ebrahim (1985)

See How They Grow — *Monitoring child growth for appropriate health care in developing countries* D Morley and M Woodland (1979) *ELBS*

Nutrition and Families J A S Ritchie (1983) *TALC*

Common Medical Problems in the Tropics C R Schull (1987) *TALC*

Guidelines to Drug Usage G Upunda, J Yudkin, G V Brown (1983) *TALC*

Sanitation Without Water U Winblad and W Kilama (1985) *TALC*

Rural Water Supply and Sanitation — *Blair Research Bulletins* P Morgan (1990)

Family Care — *How to look after yourself and your family* M Skeet (1981)

Macmillan Family Health Guide in the Tropics (1987)

Macmillan Human Biology Wallcharts — *Ten colour wallcharts* (1989)

The Family Planning Clinic in Africa R Brown and J Brown (1988) *TALC*

Preventing a Crisis — *AIDS and family planning work* G Gordon and T Klouda (1989) *Co-published with IPPF*

The AIDS Handbook J Hubley (1990)

First Aid in Illness and Injury M Skeet (1990)

Hanyane — *A village struggles for eye health* E Sutter, A Foster and V Francis (1989)

Maternal and Child Health in Practice G J Ebrahim, A Ahmed, A Khan (1988) *TALC*

Nutrition in Mother and Child Health G J Ebrahim (1983) *TALC*

Paediatric Practice in Developing Countries G J Ebrahim (1981) *ELBS*

Practical Mother and Child Health — *4th Edition* G J Ebrahim (1991) *ELBS*

Breastfeeding: *The biological option 2nd Edition* G J Ebrahim (1991) *ELBS*

Puppets for Better Health G Gordon and S Gordon (1986)

Child-to-Child A Aarons (1981)

Children's Illnesses in Warm Climates J Llewellyn (1987)

Community Health Care *(Macmillan Tropical Nursing and Health Sciences Series)* A Adegoroye (1984)

TALC denotes low cost books published in association with Teaching Aids at Low Cost.

ELBS denotes subsidised English Language Book Society editions.

TEACHING HEALTH-CARE WORKERS

A Practical Guide

FRED ABBATT
and
ROSEMARY McMAHON

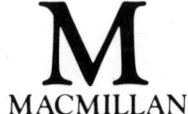
MACMILLAN

© Copyright text Fred Abbatt and Rosemary McMahon 1985

All rights reserved. No reproduction, copy or transmission of
this publication may be made without written permission.

No paragraph of this publication may be reproduced, copied or
transmitted save with written permission or in accordance with
the provisions of the Copyright, Designs and Patents Act 1988,
or under the terms of any licence permitting limited copying
issued by the Copyright Licensing Agency, 90 Tottenham Court Road,
London W1P 9HE.

Any person who does any unauthorised act in relation to this
publication may be liable to criminal prosecution and civil
claims for damages.

First published 1985
Reprinted 1988, 1989, 1990, 1991 (twice)

Published by THE MACMILLAN PRESS LTD
London and Basingstoke
*Associated companies and representatives in Accra,
Auckland, Delhi, Dublin, Gaborone, Hamburg, Harare,
Hong Kong, Kuala Lumpur, Lagos, Manzini, Melbourne,
Mexico City, Nairobi, New York, Singapore, Tokyo.*

ISBN 0-333-38614-0

Printed in Malaysia by
Chee Leong Press Sdn. Bhd.

A catalogue record for this book is available from
the British Library.

CONTENTS

	Foreword	xi
	How to Use this Book	xiii
	Acknowledgements	xv

1 Primary Health Care: What does it Mean? ... 1

- 1.1 Origins ... 2
- 1.2 The Changed Meaning of Primary Health Care ... 3
- 1.3 The Limitations of 'Medical Care' ... 4
- 1.4 The World Health Organization and Primary Health Care ... 5
- 1.5 Primary Health Care—Definition, Principles, Strategies and Elements ... 6
- 1.6 The two Sides of the 'Health Coin'—Medical Care and Primary Health Care ... 9
- 1.7 What are the Special Features of Teaching Primary Health Care? ... 9

2 The Job of the Teacher ... 15

- 2.1 What is a Teacher? ... 15
- 2.2 Deciding what Students Should Learn ... 17
- 2.3 Helping the Students to Learn ... 18
- 2.4 Checking that Learning has Occurred ... 20
- 2.5 Taking Responsibility for Students' Welfare ... 21
- 2.6 The Teacher as a Member of a Health Team ... 22

3 Deciding what should be Learnt—An Overview ... 27

- 3.1 What should be the Overall Aim of a Course? ... 27
- 3.2 What are the Consequences of Preparing Students to do a Job? ... 28
- 3.3 Finding out about the Job ... 30
- 3.4 Writing down the Job as a List of Tasks ... 34
- 3.5 How much Detail should be Given? ... 35
- 3.6 Conclusion ... 36

4 How to Write a List of Tasks for a Training Course in Primary Health Care ... 39

- 4.1 Making the Draft List of Tasks for your Course ... 39
- 4.2 Improving the Draft List of Tasks by Considering Curricula, Job Descriptions and Manuals ... 42

4.3	Improving the Task List by Comparing it with the Health Needs of the Community	45
4.4	Improving the Task List by Observing a Health Worker at Work	47
4.5	Conclusion	48

5 Examples of Tasks Performed by Primary Health Care Workers — 51

5.1	Who Performs Primary Health Care Tasks?	51
5.2	The Tasks of the Primary Health Care Worker	51
5.3	The Problem-solving Process	54
5.4	A Classification of Problem-solving Tasks Related to Primary Health Care Elements	55
5.5	Examples of Tasks Related to Primary Health Care Elements	55

6 Task Analysis — 61

6.1	Why is Task Analysis Useful?	61
6.2	What do we Mean by a Task Analysis?	63
6.3	How to do a Task Analysis	64
6.4	Defining Relevant and Necessary Knowledge	69
6.5	Conclusion	71

7 Planning the Teaching — 73

7.1	Grouping the Task List	73
7.2	Planning a Course Programme	74
7.3	Why is it Important to Plan a Course Programme?	74
7.4	How to Plan a Course Programme	75
7.5	Example of a Course Programme	76
7.6	Planning a Lesson	77
7.7	Planning Practical Work and Field Visits	83
7.8	Review	84

8 Planning the Assessment — 87

8.1	What is Assessment?	87
8.2	Why is Assessment Necessary?	87
8.3	Some Consequences for Assessment	88
8.4	Features of Effective Assessment	90
8.5	Some Issues in Organising Assessment	92
8.6	Some Assessment Methods	94
8.7	The Objective Structured Practical Examination (OSPE)	94

9 Learning Principles and Teaching Techniques — 105

9.1	Learning Principles	105
9.2	Wanting to Learn—Motivation	105
9.3	Social Relationships	107
9.4	Physical Environment	107

9.5	Clarity	108
9.6	Relevance to the Future	109
9.7	Relevance to Previous Experience	109
9.8	Structure	110
9.9	Active Learning	112
9.10	Feedback	113
9.11	Speed	113
9.12	Some Methods for Improving Clarity and Structure	114
9.13	Handouts and Manuals	115
9.14	Some Methods for Encouraging Active Participation	115

10 Teaching and Assessing Knowledge — 121

10.1	What do we Mean by 'Knowledge'	121
10.2	The Importance of Knowledge	122
10.3	The Functions of a Teacher in Helping Students Acquire Knowledge	123
10.4	Selecting Relevant and Necessary Knowledge	123
10.5	Establishing Sources of Information	126
10.6	Helping Students to Learn the Knowledge	128
10.7	Presenting Information Effectively	128
10.8	Helping Students to Remember Facts	132
10.9	Helping Students to Refer to Information Sources	133
10.10	Assessing Knowledge	134
10.11	Oral Examinations	135
10.12	Written Examinations	136
10.13	Open Book Examinations	140

11 Teaching and Assessing Attitudes — 143

11.1	What are Attitudes?	143
11.2	Are Attitudes Important?	144
11.3	Can Attitudes be Taught?	145
11.4	What Attitudes should be Taught?	146
11.5	Methods of Teaching Attitudes	146
11.6	Telling Students about Attitudes	147
11.7	Encouraging Students to Discuss Attitudes	148
11.8	Providing Information and Experience	149
11.9	Providing Role Models and Examples	150
11.10	Using Role-play Exercises	151
11.11	Some Examples of Role Plays	154
11.12	Assessing Attitudes	154

12 Teaching and Assessing Communication Skills — 159

12.1	What are Communication Skills?	160
12.2	The General Method of Teaching Communication Skills	163
12.3	Analysing Communication Skills	163
12.4	Describing and Demonstrating Communication Skills	164
12.5	Providing Practice in Performing Communication Skills	165
12.6	Group Discussions	166

12.7	Role Play	170
12.8	Field Experience/Interviews	172
12.9	Written Communication—Project Work	173
12.10	Assessing Communication Skills	174

13 Teaching and Assessing Manual Skills — 179

13.1	What are Manual Skills?	179
13.2	General Methods of Teaching Manual Skills	180
13.3	Deciding what Skills should be Learnt	180
13.4	Describing and Demonstrating the Manual Skill	181
13.5	Providing Initial Experience in Each Skill	182
13.6	Arranging for Further Experience	186
13.7	Assessing whether Students have Learnt the Manual Skills	193

14 Teaching and Assessing Decision-making Skills — 199

14.1	What is Meant by Decision-making Skills?	199
14.2	What are the Skills of Decision Making?	201
14.3	General Methods of Teaching Decision-making Skills	202
14.4	Analysing the Decision-making Skills	202
14.5	Describing and Demonstrating the Skills to the Learner	203
14.6	Providing Practice in Decision Making	203
14.7	Brain-storming	205
14.8	Snowballing	207
14.9	Case Histories, Case Studies and Patient-management Problems	209
14.10	Flowcharts	211
14.11	Games and Simulations	212
14.12	Role-play Exercises	213
14.13	Observed Field Work	213
14.14	Field Work with a Supervisor	214
14.15	Assessing Decision-making Skills	214

15 Evaluation of the Course — 217

15.1	What is the Teacher's Role in Evaluation?	218
15.2	What can be Evaluated?	219
15.3	How to Evaluate the Plan	219
15.4	How to Evaluate the Process	221
15.5	How to Evaluate the Product	228

Appendix 1	Resources for Primary Health Care Teachers	231
	1.A International Agencies which Supply Primary Health Care Resources	231
	1.B Selected Books and Manuals Related to Primary Health Care	233

Appendix 2	Procedures	237
Appendix 3	Continuing Education	239
Appendix 4	An Example of an Assessment Scheme	243

Index   247

Foreword

The concept of primary health care in the mid-1980s is very different from what it was 30 years ago. No longer primarily concerned with treating the sick, primary health care is not general practice or curative care with a few immunisations and some health teaching taken to the people. Primary health care depends on community involvement and participation, not only in carrying out the programme, but in the planning and preparation for it.

If primary health care is so different from our old concepts of medical care then we also need a very different teaching from that which is offered to, say, medical students or postgraduates. This teaching covers new and very different ground. It is also very difficult to provide as those who are taught will not just be using technologies to treat or prevent illnesses. They will be also working with the community to change the whole background in which these occur. This book is not concerned so much with teaching the actual part-time or village health worker, who so often is illiterate or semi-literate. Rather it is aiming to teach those who will be the local team-leaders of these village health workers—the medical assistants, nurses, or whatever they are called in different countries.

Fred Abbatt and Rosemary McMahon are ideally suited to write this. Few can bring so much experience. Fred Abbatt for the last 6 years has been running the highly successful course at Liverpool to train teachers of primary health care workers. Running such a course he has been in contact with such workers from around the world. He has also worked with WHO, The British Council and the UK Overseas Development Administration in many countries. This work has involved training teachers and the development of teaching programmes for health workers.

Rosemary McMahon was employed by WHO to help develop several auxiliary training programmes in Tanzania where, since independence, emphasis has been put on the training of medical assistants as the backbone of their health service. She also assisted in the development of the Rural Health series of manuals for auxiliaries published by AMREF, has worked as a consultant for World Bank funded health programmes in several countries, and has recently developed a national training programme for Community Health Officers in Sierra Leone.

This book emphasises the new knowledge and understanding of the learning process. For me it was one of the first books that I have read that has gone into, in detail, the training of the attitudes of the workers as well as detail as to how to train workers in the necessary communication skills, decision-making skills and knowledge to provide health care.

Introduction of the methods suggested in this book will lead to a dramatic change and, I believe, improvement in the training of all levels of paramedical workers. Perhaps this success will lead to the adoption of some of these methods in the training of medical students where perhaps the need for such training is equally as great.

Although aimed primarily at teachers in less-developed countries, there will be real value in this book to teachers in the West. Probably few books put so concisely how to develop the methods of designing course programmes, teaching the programmes and evaluating their success. Rosemary McMahon and Fred Abbatt are to be congratulated on their very real contribution to bringing in 'Health for all by 2000'.

London, 1985

David Morley
Professor of Child Health
Institute of Child Health

How to Use this Book

This book is a result of the authors' concern and involvement in the teaching of health-care workers in many countries. Whilst dramatic changes are taking place in the numbers of health workers trained and in the type of health care being provided, the type of training offered has not changed sufficiently. Often, the training emphasises the learning of detailed facts. The practical work and field experience may be poorly supervised and sometimes ineffective.

The aim of this book is to help teachers to rethink their whole approach to training and so to overcome these criticisms. The first two chapters describe the background of primary health care (a policy which has been adopted in nearly every country) and the role of the teacher.

Chapters 3 to 6 explain how teachers can be much more precise about what they want their students to learn. The technique of 'task analysis' is suggested which leads to clear distinctions between the different types of things which must be learnt, the knowledge and attitudes, the skills of communication and decision-making, the manual or psychomotor skills.

This definition of what needs to be learnt provides the basis for planning overall course programmes, planning the assessment of students and choosing teaching methods. These processes are described in chapters 7, 8 and 9.

The teaching methods which are most appropriate for each of the five areas of learning are then described with specific examples in chapters 10 to 14, with a final chapter on evaluating courses.

This book will not mean that teachers will be able to spend less time in teaching or that their work will be easier; rather, the authors hope that teachers will find their work more satisfying and more varied, that their students will learn more quickly and that the students will be equipped to provide a better quality of health care.

Liverpool and Sierra Leone, 1985　　　　　　　　　　　　　　　　　　F. A.
　　　　　　　　　　　　　　　　　　　　　　　　　　　　　　　　　　R. McM.

TALC

Acknowledgements

The authors and publishers would like to express their thanks and appreciation to Chris Butler for drawing most of the illustrations.

The authors and publishers wish to thank the following who have kindly given permission for the use of copyright material:

Basil Blackwell Ltd for a graph from *The Role of Medicine* by Thomas McKeown.
The MEDEX Group, University of Hawaii, for an illustration from *The MEDEX Primary Health Care Series: Clean Home and Clean Community*.
World Health Organization for the illustration 'Visiting the Community' by J. A. Halstead from *On Being in Charge: A Guide for Middle-level Management in Primary Health Care* by R. McMahon, E. Barton and M. Piot (WHO, 1980).

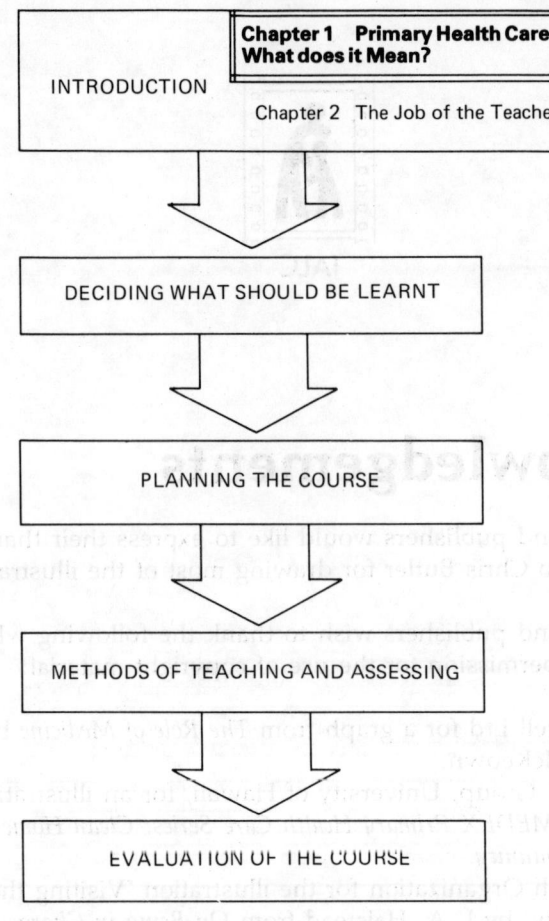

CONTENTS

1.1	Origins	2
1.2	The Changed Meaning of Primary Health Care	3
1.3	The Limitations of 'Medical Care'	4
1.4	The World Health Organization and Primary Health Care	5
1.5	Primary Health Care: Definition; Principles; Strategies; Elements	6
1.6	The Two Sides of the 'Health Coin' — Medical Care and Primary Health Care	9
1.7	What are the Special Features of Teaching Primary Health Care?	9

1
Primary Health Care: What does it mean?

'The village had changed during the past 10 years—and a major reason for the change was the Primary Health Care Programme.

The heart of the Primary Health Care programme was the village. A village health committee had chosen their own village health worker who had been trained for 6 months. She had learnt something about diseases, how they could be treated and how they could be prevented. She had also learnt how to teach in the community, so now there was a 'family health worker' in every family.

She also learnt that health is not something isolated, but closely related to other types of development. She had learnt about grain storage so that more of the food harvested was protected from the various pests and was available for the villagers to eat or sell.

She had learnt about protection of water supplies and methods of sanitation, which had been implemented by the village. She had learnt about starting micro-businesses and about making ointments and medicines from the locally available plants. So now the village people made and sold their own soap and medicines.

She had learnt about team building and organisational skills. So now the village were making their own decisions about the kind of health care they wanted and were able to identify some of the resources and people which would be useful to them.

All this activity and development had led to a reduced infant mortality rate and much lower incidence of the communicable diseases. It has also led to a community which was much more in control of its own future.'

This village does exist. It is a real place where many of the ideas of Primary Health Care (PHC) have been put into practice. So it illustrates some of the things which PHC workers can do and illustrates in practical terms what 'Primary Health Care' means.

However, in other places a policy of 'Primary Health Care' has led to rather different results. So this chapter will explain how the meaning of PHC has changed over the years and what it now means.

The development of a variety of ideas, which are now part of the PHC concept, has taken place rapidly during the past thirty years. Because ideas and programmes have changed so fast, there is widespread confusion concerning many aspects of this approach to health. This confusion affects the goals and planning undertaken by national governments and voluntary agencies. The same confusion spreads into the teaching and training of health workers and affects those who supervise and implement the programmes.

Teachers who are training health workers need to understand clearly what is meant by the PHC approach and also to see their work as part of a broad international development.

This chapter explains briefly the many elements which are now an accepted part of the PHC approach and outlines why teaching PHC has a different emphasis from teaching hospital care workers and requires special skills.

1.1 ORIGINS

Primary Health Care originally meant the *first* care given to a patient in need. In this sense every traditional 'medicine man' gives PHC and so does every doctor working in general practice in Europe and elsewhere.

Until the 1950s and beyond, and even now in some places, PHC was understood in this sense. It was an *extension* of basic medical curative services into rural or underdoctored areas.

To extend some curative services into underprivileged areas where there were few doctors or hospitals, various types of 'auxiliary health worker' were trained and placed in outlying dispensaries or treatment centres.

The idea of training auxiliary health workers has a long history. Feldshers were trained in Russia at the end of the 19th century. Auxiliary workers existed during the colonial epoch, for example, 'tribal dressers' in the British colonies in Africa and 'sub-assistant surgeons' of India.

But in the 1950s and 1960s there was a rapid expansion of these cadres and many types of worker were trained and variously named, for example, dressers, dispensers, orderlies and rural aides. These workers usually had a few years of primary schooling before a period of training. They were provided with a few simple drugs in their outposts and treated patients who came to see them.

At the same time, a more elaborate training of secondary school leavers created another class of auxiliary health worker—usually called medical assistants or clinical assistants. These auxiliaries were originally trained to work strictly under the supervision of doctors in hospitals, outpatients and urban clinics. Later, in the 1960s when the health centre idea became popular, these health workers were seen as 'team leaders' and placed in charge of health centres. At this period some preventive functions were added to their mainly curative work.

Many countries, unable to train special auxiliary workers, posted hospital trained nurses into health centres and outlying dispensaries. In this situation they necessarily assumed the function of prescribing as well as administering treatment, a new role and responsibility for which they often received no additional training.

An unspoken assumption during this period of PHC was the idea of 'substitution' or 'second best'. The ideal was seen as treatment by a doctor or in a hospital, but where this ideal was unobtainable, the common conditions could be treated by an auxiliary. This assumption and the resulting accusation of 'second class medicine' cannot be accepted now because the curative medical model itself has been challenged and the *whole meaning of PHC has changed.* As will be seen, the auxiliary is no longer seen as a substitute for a doctor but as an essential, indispensable agent of health promotion. In the new concept of PHC the auxiliary is the *key* person. He does not substitute and there is no substitute for him!

1.2 THE CHANGED MEANING OF PRIMARY HEALTH CARE

The concept of PHC now (1984) is very different indeed from the original idea of treating the sick. What is the change? and what has brought it about?

It is now recognised that 'medical care' is different from 'health care'.

The medical care model of doctors and hospitals, auxiliaries and dispensaries helps individuals who reach them after they have become ill. On the other hand, the health care model finds ways and means to prevent disease and promote health in families and communities and attempts to reduce the total amount of sickness. To give a simple example, a dispenser could live in a village for ten years and treat all the cases of hookworm which came to him but there would still remain the same level of hookworm infection because the source of the infection had not been removed and even his treated patients would be liable to reinfection. A PHC worker, on the other hand, would not be content with only treating hookworm but would actively promote sanitary changes within the community to reduce the level of transmission.

Some of this new understanding—that 'health promotion' is different from 'disease-treating'—came through studies of the history of disease in Europe.

The pattern of disease in Europe in past centuries was very similar to that in many developing countries today. Europe had epidemics of cholera and plague which killed large numbers of people, typhoid was endemic, tuberculosis rampant and there was a high infant mortality from measles, malnutrition, diarrhoea and whooping cough.

All of these conditions are no longer common in Europe. But this improvement was not brought about by medical treatment with drugs.

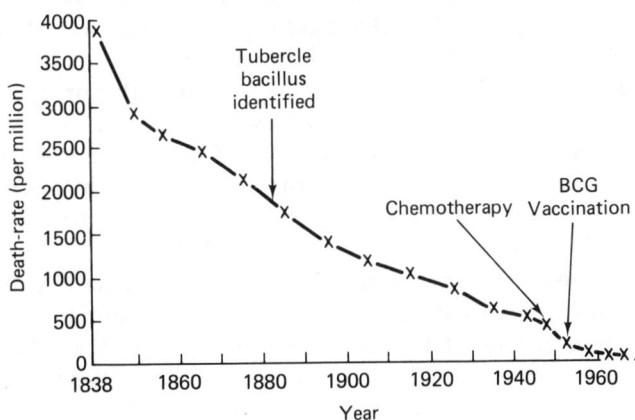

Figure 1.1 Respiratory Tuberculosis: mean annual death-rates (standardised to 1901 population): England and Wales. (Reproduced from McKeown, T. (1979) *The Role of Medicine*, Blackwell, Oxford.)

Health statistics show that reduced incidence of infectious diseases and lowered infant mortality rates occurred *before* the discovery of chemotherapy, antibiotics and most vaccines.

This is shown in figure 1.1 for tuberculosis. Mortality from respiratory tuberculosis fell sharply from the time when it was first recorded, even though the first effective treatment was only introduced in 1947 and BCG vaccination started in 1953.

The dramatic improvement of health status in Europe followed the introduction of clean water supplies, sanitation, and education (which brought the practice of hygiene into family life).

> A good clean environment brings health to people

1.3 THE LIMITATIONS OF 'MEDICAL CARE'

There were many other reasons for dissatisfaction with the 'medical model' of care and the development of the PHC concept. The first was economic. The training of doctors and the provision of hospital facilities began to drain the budgets of developing nations. It was recognised to be economically impossible to provide sufficient doctors and hospitals for all the population—even if this were desirable. Also, many highly proficient indigenous doctors became increasingly dissatisfied with inadequate facilities and migrated to the developed world. This phenomenon, now called the 'brain drain', increased the shortage of doctors in developing countries.

A further cause of dissatisfaction was that the more medical science developed, the less appropriate it became to the basic needs of people in the developing world. The increasingly specialised and sophisticated technologies practised in urban teaching hospitals were recognised by many as irrelevant to the health needs of most of the population. For example, only a few people need kidney dialysis or neurosurgery but millions of children need measles immunisation.

Another change in thought followed the development of drug resistance in some bacteria and parasites. Many drugs which were active against the malarial parasite, for example, chloroquin and pyremethamine, are now ineffective in certain parts of the world. Many common bacteria are now resistant to penicillin. This has brought the realisation that drugs may be only a short term solution. These serious developments, together with the inflation of drug prices in the Western world, have compelled health planners to search for other solutions—that is, solutions which place less dependence on short term curative effects and emphasise the preventive aspects of health care.

For all these reasons, and many others, it became clear that the 'medical care model' was not only uneconomic but was also inappropriate to the major health problems of the Third World. Some of the differences between medical care and PHC are summarised in section 1.5 of this chapter.

Persons concerned with the health of people started looking for alternative ways of care. In this search the World Health Organization played a leading role. And it was during this search that many ideas were formulated and tried out. Many of these new ways to improve health became included in the idea of PHC—and in this way, the words changed their meaning.

Some of these ideas which now form the PHC approach are explained below.

> Primary Health Care is more than medical care

1.4 THE WORLD HEALTH ORGANIZATION AND PRIMARY HEALTH CARE

A new interest in health followed the end of the colonial empires, the rise of independent governments and the awakening of people to their 'rights' and 'needs'.

The World Health Organization both reflected and channelled this growing demand for improved health. This culminated in the idea initiated by the Director General of WHO, Dr H. Mahler in 1975 which was expressed later in the now famous slogan

> Health for all by the year 2000

The resolution in which the nations of the world voted to work for this goal was passed by the 30th World Health Assembly in May 1977.

This resolution was rapidly followed by an international conference at Alma Ata (January 1978) which discussed PHC as one of the ways to bring about this goal of Health for All. This conference brought together

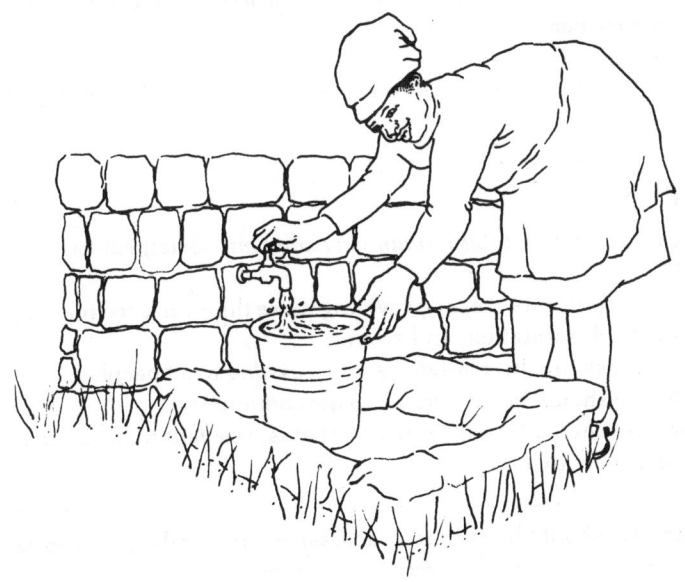

Figure 1.2 Health care includes providing a supply of clean water. (Reproduced from *The Medex Primary Health Care Series: Clean Home and Clean Community*, Johns A. Burns School of Medicine, Hawaii, U.S.A.)

many of the ideas and experience of the past thirty years and explained in a clear document the principles, strategies and elements of the PHC approach. At present, this approach is regarded by the World Health Organization as the most suitable road to follow towards the goal of universal health.

The PHC complex of ideas is by no means completed. Further strategies are even now developing—in particular, ideas of using community evaluation as a motivator to action and methods by which health care can be partially self-financing.

Primary Health Care is not a package. It is not a finished, complete, defined methodology. Rather, it is a *process* or an approach which grows as our understanding of human development increases.

> Primary Health Care is an approach to achieve health for all

1.5 PRIMARY HEALTH CARE—DEFINITION, PRINCIPLES, STRATEGIES AND ELEMENTS

Definition

The following is the definition of PHC which emerged from the Alma Ata Conference.

> 'Primary Health Care is essential health care based on practical, scientifically sound and socially acceptable methods and technology, made universally accessible to individuals and families in the community through their full participation and at a cost the community and country can afford to maintain at every stage of their development in the spirit of self-reliance and self-determination.'

As will be seen many of the basic principles of PHC are included in this definition.

Principles

Health care is part of *total human development*, social, educational and economic.

Essential health care means providing those things needed for a healthy life, water, food, sanitation, and so on.

Health care should be *available* and *accessible* to all people.

Health care should be *acceptable* to the community.

Health care should be *appropriate*—that is, relevant to the main health problems of an area.

> Health care should be available, accessible, acceptable, appropriate

Some Strategies of Primary Health Care

Below are listed some of the ways and means used in implementing PHC and achieving the goal of health for all.

Intersectoral co-operation. Primary Health Care programmes should be set in a context of integrated development—housing, transport, agriculture, communications, education and others.

The prevention of disease and the promotion of health are essential activities in PHC.

Basic infrastructure. Some basic health facility should be established within reach of every family. This distance will depend on terrain, roads and available transport, but an acceptable average walking distance is usually taken to be 5 kilometres.

Referral system. The health facilities need to be connected through a referral mechanism to the hospital service.

Auxiliary health workers need to be trained to work in the health facilities.

Village health workers need to be trained to work in the community.

Traditional medical systems. Research is needed into the effectiveness of some traditional remedies. Training of traditional birth attendants is proving successful. Co-operation with and training of other traditional medical workers should be encouraged.

Health education is fundamental to PHC. Only through understanding the basis of a healthy life, can people make rational decisions concerning their needs and life style.

Community participation. Each community should be involved in the PHC service through the functioning of an active responsible health committee.

Health care should be *relevant* to the main health problems of each community.

Essential drugs for treating common conditions should be provided.

Cost effective and self-reliant. As a country and community develops, the provision of health care should grow. That is, the level of health care should reflect the total development and be within the means of the community.

The Eight Elements of Primary Health Care

The World Health Organization has defined eight elements of PHC. Not all of these elements are present in every health care programme. They represent a goal to work towards. As many of these elements as possible should be encouraged in every community striving towards health for all. These elements are;

Health Education	Water and Sanitation
Nutrition	Control of Endemic Diseases
Immunisation	Treatment of Common Diseases
Maternal and Child Health and Family Planning	Provision of Essential Drugs

Some of the PHC tasks related to these elements are listed in chapter 5.

Figure 1.3 shows these elements arranged as 10 components in a circle. The circle indicates that these elements are not separate from each other. They interrelate. For example, nutrition and immunisation are essential elements in the health of mothers and children. Health education is *central to all components*. Also note that treatment is only one part of health care.

We have looked briefly at the principles, strategies and elements of PHC as they have been developed over the years in the international world. It is important to realise that the way in which these are applied will be different for every country. Primary Health Care is an *approach*. It is a flexible system which needs to fit all types of circumstances. It must be adapted to the health problems, the culture, the way of life and stage of development reached by the community. Primary Health Care needs to develop as the community develops. It is part of the whole social development process.

> Primary Health Care is an approach to health

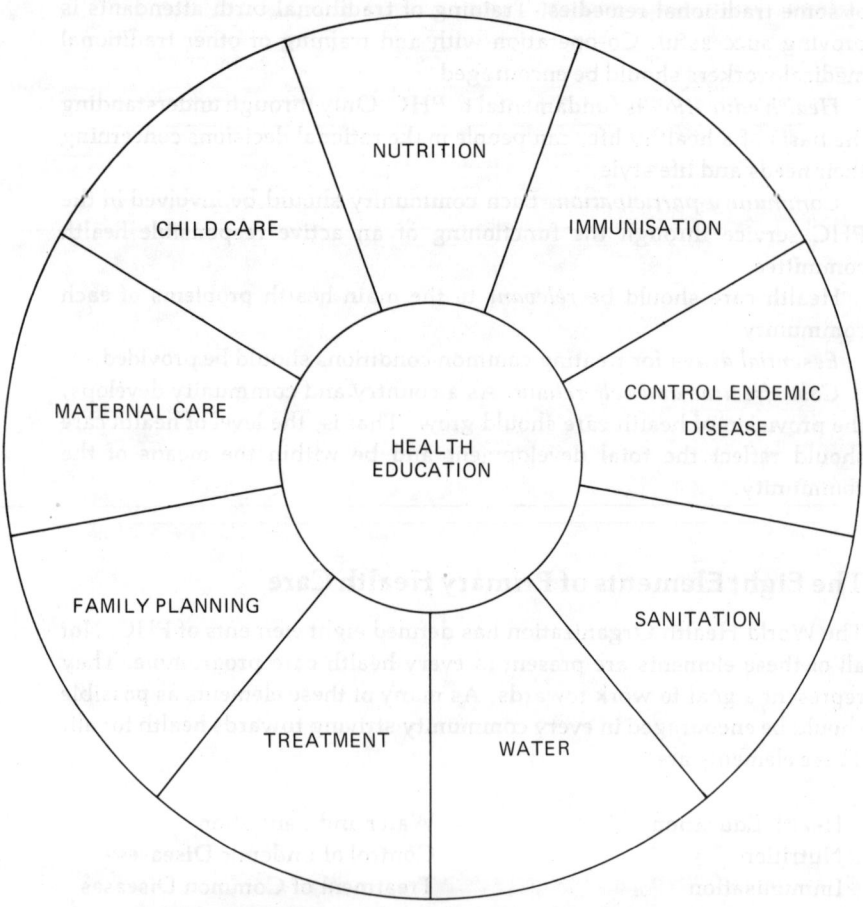

Figure 1.3   The circle of Primary Health Care

1.6 THE TWO SIDES OF THE 'HEALTH COIN'—MEDICAL CARE AND PRIMARY HEALTH CARE

We have seen that PHC is different from medical care. It has a wider range of components (water, nutrition and so on) and many different strategies (community participation and intersectoral co-operation).

But both systems of care are necessary and complement each other. A PHC worker needs to refer some patients to treatment centres or to a hospital for more specialised medical care. These two systems are best seen as two sides of a coin. Every country needs both systems of care.

Some of the differences between the two systems are summarised in table 1.1.

Table 1.1

The Medical Care system	The Primary Health Care approach
The medical system is 'vertical', i.e. separate from other government departments	This functions best through intersectoral co-operation
A curative system, emphasising treatment and drugs, doctors and hospitals or auxiliaries and dispensaries	Mainly preventive and promotive. Emphasises water, sanitation, immunisation, nutrition and health education
Emphasises improved technology and specialisation	Emphasises common conditions, 'at risk groups' and reduction of infant mortality
Treats individuals who are sick	Helps healthy people in the community to prevent sickness as well as treating the sick
Auxiliaries are regarded as substitutes for doctors	Auxiliaries are the main agents of health promotion and change
Health is seen as a technology brought in from outside	Health promotion is a family and community activity
Discourages traditional medicine and ignores culture	Encourages the health positive aspects of traditional medicine and culture
Is expensive, with a strong bias towards urban areas and hospitals	Is less expensive with a bias towards equal distribution, rural areas and the urban poor
Often paid for by central government finance	Partly supported by community self-reliance
Causes the patient to be dependent on the doctor, nurse and health service	Helps the individuals and communities to become more capable of looking after themselves

1.7 WHAT ARE THE SPECIAL FEATURES OF TEACHING PRIMARY HEALTH CARE?

In the previous sections of this chapter we have explained some of the ideas concerning PHC which are current in the world at the present time. These ideas have been developed by the World Health Organization in co-operation with national governments. But it is recognised that for the implementation of these ideas well-trained PHC workers are essential.

Because PHC differs in many ways from hospital-based curative care, the training of PHC workers needs to be different from that of nurses and hospital auxiliaries.

Below we outline five features which we think need special emphasis in the training of PHC workers. Because of these features teachers of PHC need to develop exceptional skills. This book is meant to help teachers understand the needs of PHC workers and develop the skills necessary to train them.

(i) The Need to Focus on 'Performance' during Training

Primary Health Care is practical work. It is what the health worker *can do* in his daily life to promote health in his community which is important. Therefore the good PHC teacher will concentrate his teaching on the *performance* of his students—what they can do and how well they can do it. Performing well is important for all health workers—but whereas hospital nurses work under continual supervision and continue learning after qualifying by on the job training, the PHC worker often works alone in isolated areas shortly after qualifying. So he has little supervision in the development of his performance skills after the initial training period.

(ii) The Need for 'Flexibility' in Training

Because PHC is a developmental approach, the system differs in each area. There are many types of PHC worker, there are courses of different lengths and depths and different systems of care in each country. There is no such thing as a standard PHC curriculum: each training programme is unique.

In this situation PHC teachers need to be flexible and to be able to adapt the content and method of training to the needs of the community and the level of the students.

(iii) The Need to Teach Decision Making

Most PHC workers are stationed alone or with one or two others in isolated rural areas. They need to be able to examine the community health situation, to make judgements concerning health priorities and decide when and how to initiate changes. As responsible health workers they are faced daily with decisions concerning the diagnosis, management or referral of patients. They need to develop an approach to decision making which is based on an appraisal of the facts of the situation combined with an assessment of community values. PHC workers need training in the basic principles of reaching decisions.

(iv) The Need to Teach 'Communication'

We believe that the most essential skill of the PHC worker is the *ability to communicate well*. This is because bringing health to people depends to a major extent on *community participation*. Primary Health Care programmes only function when communities and families *actively participate* in changing some aspects of the environment and habits of life. This active participation is dependent on the PHC worker being effective in communicating health-promoting messages to the community.

The factor of active community participation is fundamental to all successful PHC programmes. Some ways in which families and communities help bring about healthy living conditions are shown in table 1.2. The advice, explanations, discussions of the PHC worker encourage people to take part in the activities which promote their health. To advise well, explain clearly, listen sympathetically and discuss fruitfully requires communication skills on the part of the health worker.

It is because the health promoting activities undertaken by the people are so dependent on the communication skills of the health worker that we believe teaching communication skills is an essential feature of PHC training.

Table 1.2 How PHC tasks need the active participation of people

	Community activities which improve health	*Family activities which improve health*	*Health-worker activities which improve health*
Nutrition	Farmers plant nutritional crops which grow well locally (e.g. beans, pulses, fruits) Farmers adopt methods which increase food yields	Mothers breast feed Family grows vegetables Mothers prepare good weaning foods	Health worker supervises a demonstration garden at the health centre Health worker encourages the planting of nutritional crops Health worker identifies nutritional deficiencies
Water	Health committee organises the protection of the local water supply Health committee maintains the pump of the community well	Family stores water in clean containers	Health worker sends water samples for testing Health worker prevents waterborne diseases by advising the community
Maternal care	Health committee encourages the training of local traditional birth attendants Community council arranges a subsidised transport system for mothers with an obstetric emergency	Mother prepares a clean room for home delivery Mother attends antenatal clinic regularly	Health worker conducts regular antenatal examinations Health worker gives prophylactic medicines during pregnancy (iron, chloroquin) Health worker detects and refers at-risk mothers

(v) The Need to Learn 'How to Learn'

Primary Health Care workers will find more interest in their work if they continue learning after qualifying and continue developing their skills. This particularly applies to those who have reached the level of secondary school education. Continued learning may be achieved through refresher courses, in-service training courses or, in some countries, upgrading courses. For this to be effective the idea of learning throughout life needs to be introduced during training. Those who learn to take pleasure in developing their skills and increasing their knowledge during training are likely to continue this pleasure after qualifying. Many manuals, journals and newsletters are available nowadays for PHC workers: some of these are listed in Appendix 1. If these are introduced during training, the health worker may carry on reading them after qualifying. Continuing education and keeping up interest are important factors in motivating

Teaching Health-Care Workers

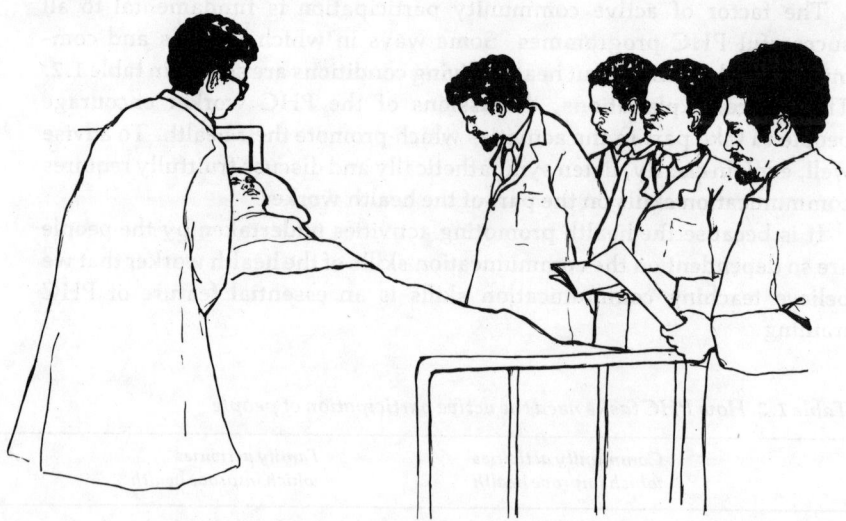

Figure 1.4 'Here I find the work very scientifically stimulating'

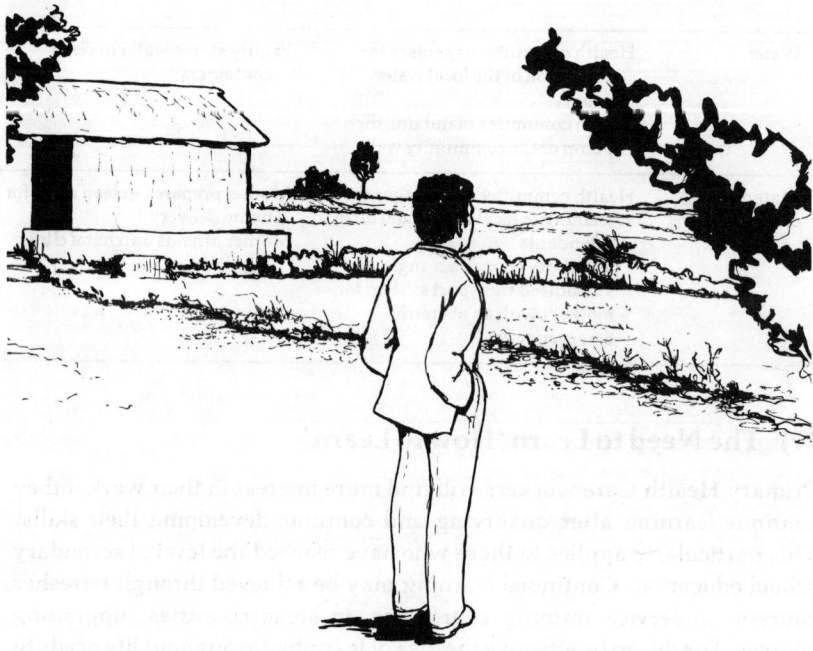

Figure 1.5 'Here I have been able to help the community improve their health'

workers—more especially those who are isolated and only occasionally receive supervisory visits.

SUMMARY
- The meaning of PHC has changed during the past 30 years.
- Primary Health Care is very different from medical care.
- Primary Health Care is seen by WHO as the strategy for achieving health for all.
- Primary Health Care is part of total development. It should be health-promoting, available, accessible, appropriate, cost-effective and self-reliant. The eight elements and various strategies are derived from these principles.
- These new concepts of PHC have implications for teaching PHC workers.

  These are: the need to emphasise performance and to be flexible in approach; the need to teach both communication and decision making as distinct skills; and the importance of helping students to learn how to learn and encouraging continued learning throughout working life.

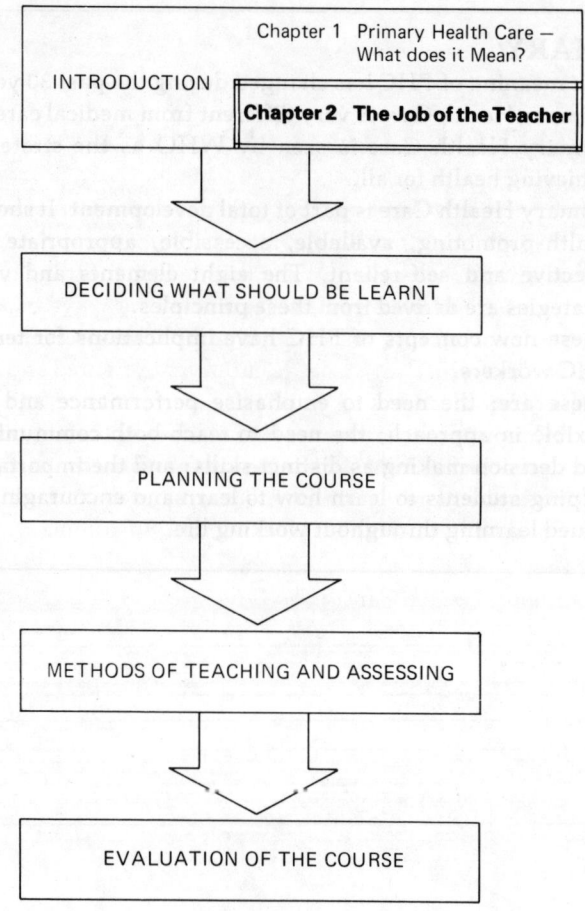

CONTENTS

2.1	What is a Teacher?	15
2.2	Deciding what Students Should Learn	17
2.3	Helping the Students to Learn	18
2.4	Checking that Learning has Occurred	20
2.5	Taking Responsibility for Students' Welfare	21
2.6	The Teacher as a Member of a Health Team	22

2
The Job of the Teacher

In the previous chapter we have outlined the modern meaning of Primary Health Care (PHC) and have explained some of the ways in which the health workers involved in PHC face quite different problems to those faced by the health workers in the more curatively-oriented and hospital-based systems of health care.

Because PHC requires different kinds of health workers, the training for these workers must be different. It must equip the worker with the skills of communication and of prevention of disease as well as curative care. Without these skills the whole PHC ideal will fail. In summary

> Effective Primary Health Care depends on effective and appropriate training

How can the teacher help to make this training effective? This chapter will start to answer this question by looking at what teachers do. This is followed by guidance on how this work can be done better and where advice on this is given in this book.

2.1 WHAT IS A TEACHER?

If you tell a new friend that you are a teacher, this friend will probably think that you spend your time in a classroom with students. The friend may also think that you have a good knowledge of a particular subject and that you spend a lot of your time telling students about this subject.

This is a fairly normal idea about what teachers are and what they do. This book will argue that an effective teacher of PHC workers does very much more than this. Some people sum up the work of a teacher by saying that they should 'manage the learning process'. Others argue that a teacher should be a 'facilitator of learning'. Both of these phrases include the key idea that teachers should help other people to learn.

> Teaching is helping other people to learn

Probably you would accept the idea that the best teachers are those whose students learn the most (provided that *what* the students learn is appropriate). However this general idea does not explain what teachers do when they are helping students to learn. Is a person who stands in a classroom talking to students actually teaching? The answer depends on whether the students learn anything. If they do, the person is teaching. If the students do not learn, then the person is just talking.

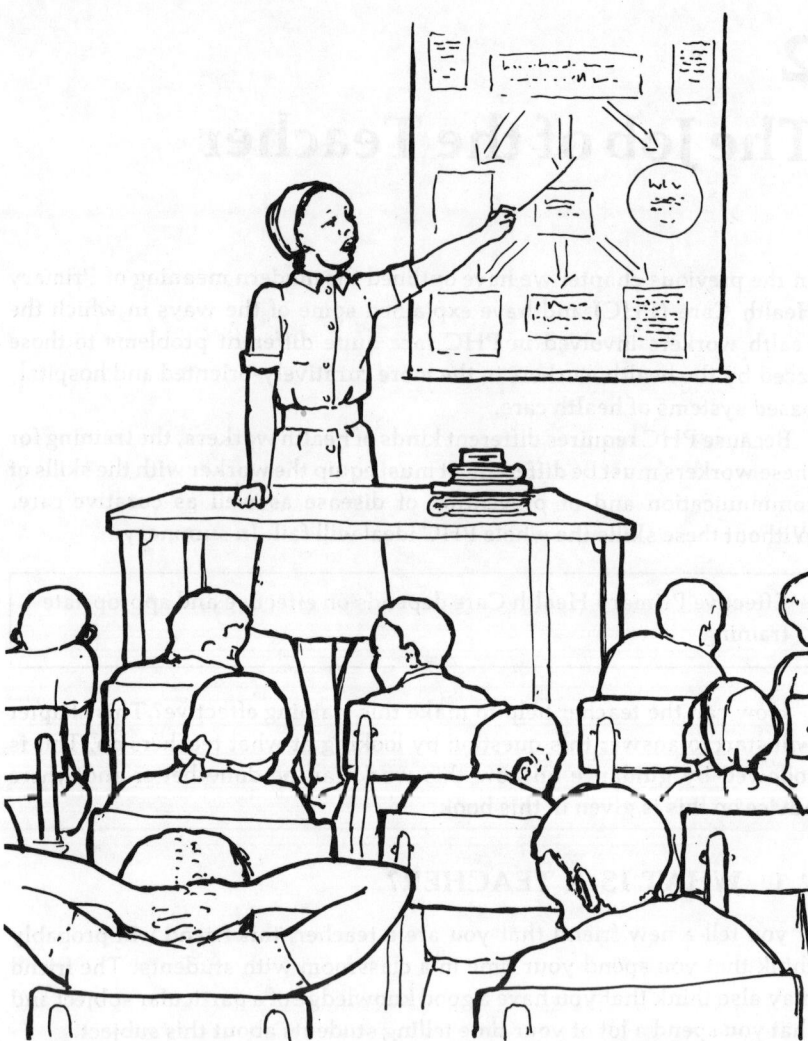

Figure 2.1 Is this teacher teaching—or is she just talking?

If a person organises students to read something in a manual, or sets the students a problem to solve, or arranges for the students to do practical work in the field—then that person is teaching. A teacher does *not* need to be providing facts all the time. In fact, much of the best teaching is done when the teacher is silent and allows the students to learn. This general idea will be discussed in much more detail later on in the book.

We have just said that teaching is not the same thing as talking—but what does it involve? Broadly, there are four general parts of the job:

(1) Deciding what students should learn.
(2) Helping the students to learn.
(3) Checking whether the students have learnt.
(4) Taking responsibility for student welfare.

These four parts are explained in the sections below.

2.2 DECIDING WHAT STUDENTS SHOULD LEARN

It is obvious that at some point in the process of teaching and learning, decisions have to be made about what the students should learn. If there is a course for orthopaedic surgeons it should be totally different to a course for health inspectors. Health inspectors do not need to be able to replace hip joints and orthopaedic surgeons do not need to control the breeding sites of mosquitoes.

The decisions about what should be included in a course and what should be left out are taken by several different groups of people: the Ministry of Health may be involved, there may be curriculum committees and the students themselves may have an important contribution to make in this decision. However, the teacher should be involved with these different groups in making the decisions. And, of course, it is the teacher who has the job of interpreting general curricula or syllabuses. It is the teacher who has to decide how much detail or depth in a particular area is appropriate. And it is the teacher who has the responsibility of explaining to students why some things are more important to learn than others.

Decisions about what should be learnt are made at very different levels of detail. An outline syllabus may be laid down by the Ministry of Health or a Board of Examiners. Many individual teachers will have very little opportunity to influence this outline. However, it is impossible to specify a course in enough detail to eliminate the need for teachers to make their own decisions. For example, if a course outline for birth attendants says that students should be able to 'cut the cord hygienically' when delivering a baby, the outline does not specify where the cut should be made, nor whether the attendant should use a razor blade or a piece of sharpened bamboo. Always the teacher will have to fill in the details.

Making decisions about what should be learnt is possibly the most important job of the teacher.

Unfortunately this very important set of decisions is often poorly made and fails to take account of work which needs to be done in PHC. As an example of what can go wrong, village health workers might be taught 'Nutrition'. At first this seems excellent. After all, nutritional deficiency is common in many places and is known to be a very important factor in the deaths of many children. So what is wrong? Well, it depends on what the health workers learn in 'Nutrition'. They might learn how the various foods are absorbed in the intestine, that different types of food have different functions, that the amount of energy (or protein) per gram of beans is so much. All of these things are reasonable and part of 'Nutrition'. But is this what the village health worker needs?

The answer is 'Yes' and 'No'! Maybe the outline suggests more details than are really necessary, but this background information is almost certainly useful. The thing that is really wrong is that the health worker may be able to write essays on nutrition, but will he be able to do anything *useful* with the knowledge? For example, will he be able to persuade a mother to change the way she weans her baby? This ability to persuade will depend partly on having the necessary knowledge about nutrition. But it will depend very much more on the health worker's skill in communication and persuasion. It may depend on the health worker's ability to cultivate suitable crops and to show other people in the village how to do this. It may depend on the health worker's attitudes, particularly his respect for the cultural patterns and traditions of the village.

If the teacher decides that what students need to learn is just the scientific or medical facts, then the course will be a disaster. Instead the teacher should always be thinking about what the learner will do in his job after the course—and this is what the teacher should be helping the students to learn.

> Courses for Primary Health Care workers should teach them how to do the job

In chapters 3, 4 and 5 these ideas will be developed and explained in more detail. We will also explain how the decisions can be made about 'what the students should learn'.

2.3 HELPING THE STUDENTS TO LEARN

Having decided what students need to learn, the second role of the teacher is to do all those things which will help the students to learn.

This is not just a fancy phrase for traditional classroom teaching and lecturing. Helping learning concentrates on what the learner does during the learning process. So, helping learning involves, for example:

- asking appropriate questions for the students to answer,
- organising exercises or simulations in which the students have to make plans and reach decisions,
- arranging experiences during which the students will apply facts or will perhaps develop attitudes,
- showing a film or photographs,
- arranging laboratory work,
- planning an experiment for the students to carry out,
- supervising students whilst they conduct a survey.

All these things are likely to help learning and are only a very small number of all the possibilities.

It cannot be emphasised too often that standing in a classroom and talking is *only one* of the ways of helping students to learn—and often not even a very good method.

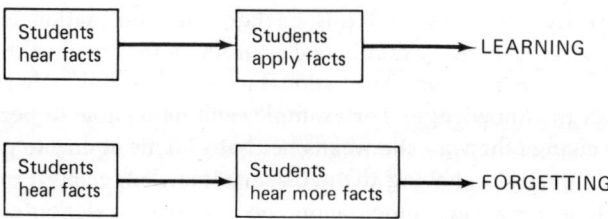

The Job of the Teacher 19

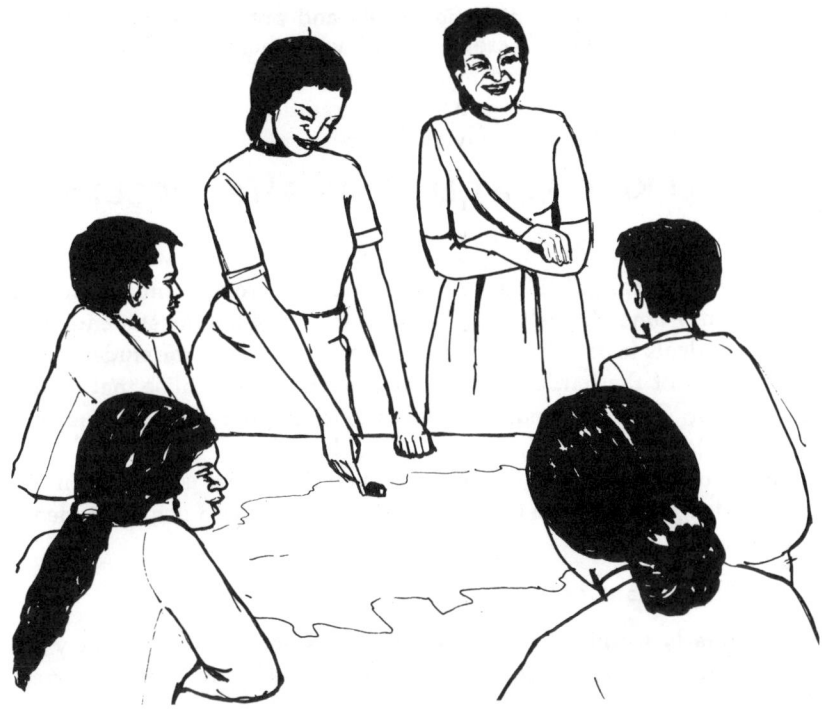

Figure 2.2 These students are learning, even though the teacher is not there

At first sight the range of teaching methods (which is much easier to write and read than 'methods of helping learning') may seem vast and confusing. It may seem as though one method is more or less as good as another method. In fact, this is not the case. There are fairly well established principles which describe in general terms what affects the speed at which people learn. For example, when students apply the facts that they learn immediately after they first learn them, these facts will be remembered very much better than if the students spend their time learning more facts.

So, if students learn some principles of communication and then go on to use these principles immediately in a role play or in a home visit, they will learn these principles much much better than if they go on to learn something different.

These principles which help you to decide which methods are likely to be most effective are described in chapter 9.

Of course one method is not best for every situation. The situation will be a very important factor in deciding which method to use. One of the most important features of the situation is the nature of what you want the students to learn. If you want the students to change their attitudes in some way, you will probably use a different teaching method to the one you would use if you want them to remember the life cycle of the round worm.

Always the teaching method should match what you want the students to learn. Chapter 6 will explain how the various things which students learn differ in their nature. It will also explain how you can classify these things. Here it may be worth reminding you that PHC requires much more emphasis on communication skills and problem solving abilities than it does on mere facts. So the teaching methods used should reflect this emphasis.

2.4 CHECKING THAT LEARNING HAS OCCURRED

When teachers are marking students' exam papers you will often hear them saying things like 'How could they get this wrong? I must have told them twenty times!'. Well, may be the teacher did tell the students; but did the students learn? Did the teacher check whether all the students had learnt? One of the hardest things for a teacher is to realise that telling students or showing students does not mean that the students will inevitably learn. Some may. Others probably will not.

Since students do not always learn everything that is covered in the course it is a vital part of a teacher's job to find out how much the students have learnt.

This is important for several reasons.

(1) Regularly testing the students tells the students how well they are getting on and where they need to spend more time to correct weaknesses.
(2) The results of the testing also tell the teacher what parts of the course have been learnt and which parts will require additional teaching—or perhaps should be taught differently in future courses.
(3) The testing will help to determine which students are suitable to work in PHC.

This checking will ideally range from the almost continuous asking of questions and observation of students whilst they do the course work through to the setting and marking of end-of-course qualifying exams.

Throughout this range of activities (which can all be called 'Assessment of students') it is important that a much wider range of methods is used than sometimes happens. Again (like methods of teaching), methods of assessment should match the ability or skill which you want to test. Whilst essays may be useful for testing students' skills in analysing problems in Philosophy, and multiple choice tests may be good at finding out which facts students know, neither of these methods will be any good at finding out whether a student can persuade a reluctant mother to breast feed instead of bottle feed.

Chapter 8 summarises the different methods of assessment and explains how they can be combined in a comprehensive plan or policy for assessment. Since assessment methods should match the kinds of abilities to be tested, the assessment methods are described in detail in chapters 10–14. These chapters consider the various types of skills and how to teach and assess them.

2.5 TAKING RESPONSIBILITY FOR STUDENTS' WELFARE

Although the major responsibility of a teacher is to help students learn a good teacher will not ignore the other aspects of his students' lives. What happens to your students outside the classroom? Do they have problems in their living conditions? Do they need some organised social events? Are they worried or lonely because they are away from home for the first time? Do they have personal problems? A teacher's responsibility for students' welfare can be considered in two aspects:
(i) Supervising students' general living conditions.
(ii) Personal counselling.

Supervising Students' General Living Conditions

How much an individual teacher can do in this respect depends on circumstances. Students may be living in an institution or they may be lodging in private houses or hostels within a town. There is a wide variety of student living situations and always there are financial limitations to the amount of assistance which can be given. Some teachers give their time outside the classroom to help students organise sporting or social events. Where this is possible it often improves relationships among the students and between students and teachers.

It is not relevant to this book to detail ways and means by which teachers can help improve the lives of students outside the classroom. The main point we wish to stress is that teachers should be aware that the conditions under which students live and the way they spend their time outside the classroom will have a profound effect on their general wellbeing and their ability to learn.

Personal Counselling

A quite different area of responsibility for teachers is counselling. Counselling has nothing to do with teaching facts or skills; instead it is concerned with helping students to deal with their learning or personal problems. Such problems might include students who are lonely or unsettled as a result of living away from their own homes for the first time; students who have poor study habits or students who have serious worries about whether they can cope with the demands of the course.

When students have serious worries or problems, they are unlikely to be able to learn very much and so it is clearly right that teachers should try to help the students to overcome their problems. This is part of being a good teacher.

This book does not set out to discuss counselling techniques—complete books on this subject alone have been written. Instead, the simple point is made that counselling is part of the job of a teacher.

2.6 THE TEACHER AS A MEMBER OF A HEALTH TEAM

The previous sections have outlined four of the major aspects of a teacher's work. What they have not done is to point out that this work is not done in isolation, but is done in collaboration with other people.

> The teacher is a member of a team

The team of which the teacher is a member, is that team bringing the PHC approach to the community. The team consists of the Ministry of Health, the local staff of the health service, the Examining Board, qualified PHC workers and, most important, the present students. The relationship of the teacher with all these people is clearly important to the success of his work.

The most important relationship is the teacher's relationship with the students. Teaching is not a battle with the students; nor should it become a struggle to maintain authority or status. Both the teachers and the students should have the same goal; that is for students to learn appropriate skills and attitudes which will help them to serve the community most effectively. So when this partnership of purpose exists, the teachers and students will discuss together what needs to be learnt and how this can best be achieved. To some extent this is idealistic. In some cultures there is a great psychological distance between teachers and students and the kind of partnership described above would seem very strange. Indeed there are some apparent advantages to a system where the teacher is very far apart from the students. For example, when teachers are remote from students, there is a fairly clear relationship and each person's responsibilities are well defined. The student hands over responsibility for his learning to the teacher and provided the student does what the teacher says he should do, then he has done what is required. It is also comfortable for the teacher. What the teacher says is not questioned or challenged in any way.

However, this kind of relationship does have rather more serious disadvantages. The students' lack of responsibility for deciding what should be learnt inevitably results in a lack of emotional involvement. Think how quickly you were able to learn something that you had decided for yourself was important to you. Think also how difficult it is to learn things that you do not really want to learn but which someone has told you should be learnt. The argument for sharing responsibility with students is also based on what happens *after* the course. Many PHC workers are posted to places of comparative isolation. Once they have been posted they often have very little supervision and so are left very much on their own. They should aim to continue learning throughout their career by observing the consequences of their own activities and by reading or listening to others. Without this continuation of their training through self-education the quality of health care cannot improve and is likely to decline. But if the students learn during training that the only source of information is the teacher or they learn that they are not competent to make their own decisions about learning, then they are very unlikely to learn in the field. On the other hand, where the teacher is in partnership with students so that students have much more responsibility, then learning will be more likely to continue throughout a career.

> Teachers should work in partnership with students

How far the teachers should hand over responsibility to students must be decided in each situation. If too much responsibility is given to students, they may not behave in a sufficiently responsible way and will waste their time and may not learn well. On the other hand, giving the students too little responsibility tends to make them behave more like young children and they will never learn to accept the very serious responsibilities involved in being a PHC worker. The ideal then is to control the amount of responsibility so that the students play an increasing role in decision making throughout the course—with the teacher always observing and checking discreetly to make sure that the students do not abuse their responsibility.

> The aim of teaching is to help the learner to become independent of the teacher

Teachers should also be in a team with the Ministry of Health and with local managers of health services. This is because the 'product' of the training programme (i.e. the students) will be employed to do a job in the health service. It is obviously important that the 'product' should be the right kind of person with the appropriate skills and beliefs. It sometimes happens that the link between training and the health system is very weak. This will be the case where teachers say things like 'This is an academic matter for teachers to decide—it is not the business of the health service'.

When this link is weak there is the obvious danger that the students who complete the training programme will be unsuitable for the work to be done. This is seen when the newly qualified health workers only want to work in towns and not in the rural areas, when they want to diagnose sitting in the health centre rather than going into the homes of people living in the community, or when they choose to spend too much of their time providing curative care rather than trying to prevent the diseases occurring.

Clearly if teachers sit down and talk with the people from the Ministry of Health or with local health care managers, this will not be enough by itself to solve all the problems. But it will help. It is right that the health system should see training programmes as being at least partly their responsibility. After all, the manager of a workforce has to make sure that the people he employs are capable of doing the job—or receive suitable training on the job to make them competent.

Again, where the balance of responsibility should be between the teacher and the health managers is very difficult to say. What is certain is that there should be at least some serious discussion with a genuine attempt to reach agreement on the kind of skills which should be learnt.

Another group with whom teachers can usefully work are the former students. These former students who have taken the course and are now working in the field are likely to be able to give very valuable advice about what parts of the course were helpful, which parts were well taught—and which were badly taught, what skills they needed to learn but were not learnt to a sufficient standard. All this information can help teachers to plan more effective courses, but the teachers will need to make a big effort to find the time to meet former students and have discussions with them.

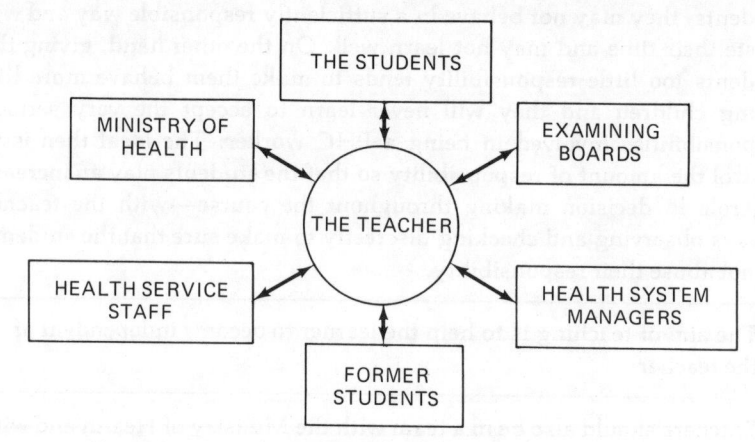

Figure 2.3   The teacher should work with other groups of people

The final group that some teachers will have to work with is the examining boards. Where courses are shorter, there may be no examining board and the teachers themselves will decide which students have passed the course and can provide health care. On the other hand, longer courses often have some kind of examining board which sets final examinations and decides what standard merits a 'pass'.

The examining boards are very powerful organisations because by means of the examination itself they determine what students will learn. (Students are unlikely to spend much time learning something which they know will not appear in the final examination.) So it is very desirable that the teachers and the examining board work together. Surprisingly the examining boards often have rather little professional training in education and so have rather limited ideas about the kind of assessment methods which are available. They tend to favour techniques like essays, multiple choice questions and oral examinations. It has already been pointed out that these techniques cannot test many of the skills needed in PHC. So it may be useful for teachers to develop new assessment methods, try them out and then let the examining boards see how they work. Obviously this will need to be done with some tact and skill!

Teachers can also work with examining boards to discuss what skills will be examined. This discussion can be based on what the teachers have learnt from former students and the managers of the health system. It can also be based on the methods of community analysis and task analysis outlined in the next chapter. In all cases the aim should be for the teachers and the examining board to establish a co-operative relationship and to agree on what they see as the important skills for students to learn and to develop appropriate techniques for assessing these skills.

> Examine skills and performance as well as knowledge

SUMMARY

In summary, the job of a teacher is to help the student to learn. This is done by:

- Deciding what the students should learn
- Helping in the learning process
- Checking that learning has occurred
- Taking responsibility for student's welfare

Throughout, the teacher should be working in partnership with students, the health system managers and examining boards (where appropriate).

Overall the teacher should help the student to become independent of the teacher by becoming capable of learning independently and capable of continuing to learn throughout his or her career in PHC

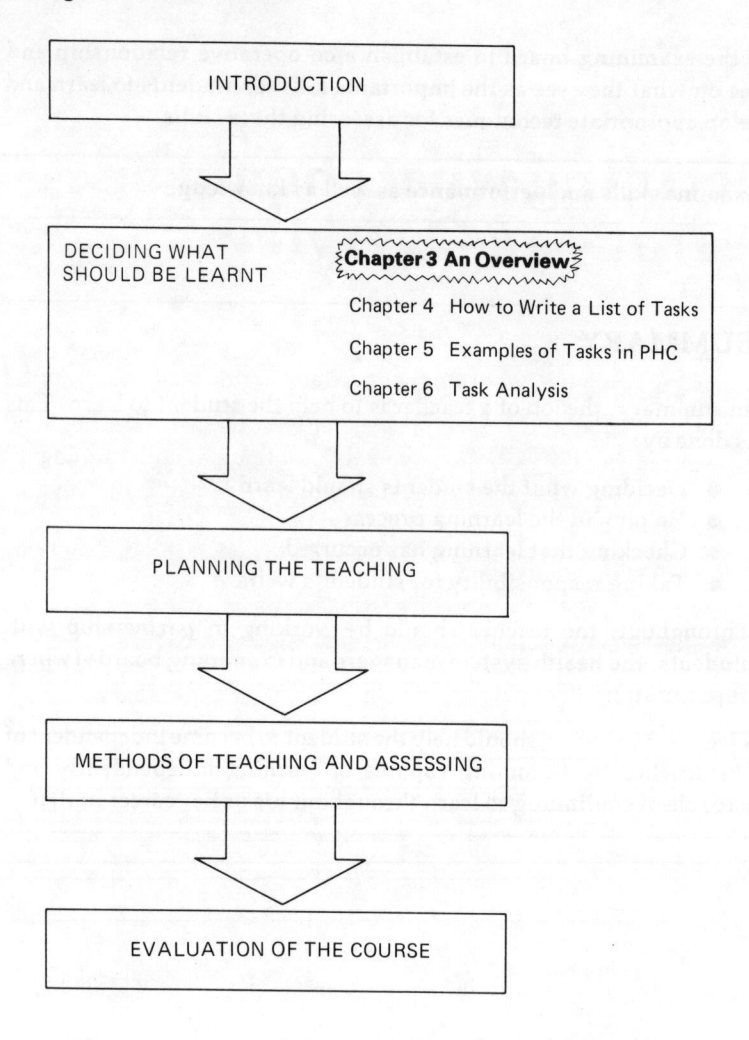

```
        ┌─────────────────────┐
        │    INTRODUCTION     │
        └─────────────────────┘
                   ↓
   ┌──────────────────────────────────────────────┐
   │ DECIDING WHAT      │ Chapter 3 An Overview    │
   │ SHOULD BE LEARNT   │                          │
   │                    │ Chapter 4  How to Write a List of Tasks │
   │                    │ Chapter 5  Examples of Tasks in PHC     │
   │                    │ Chapter 6  Task Analysis  │
   └──────────────────────────────────────────────┘
                   ↓
        ┌─────────────────────┐
        │ PLANNING THE TEACHING│
        └─────────────────────┘
                   ↓
        ┌─────────────────────────────┐
        │ METHODS OF TEACHING AND ASSESSING │
        └─────────────────────────────┘
                   ↓
        ┌─────────────────────┐
        │ EVALUATION OF THE COURSE │
        └─────────────────────┘
```

CONTENTS

3.1	What should be the Overall Aim of a Course?	27
3.2	What are the Consequences of Preparing Students to do a Job?	28
3.3	Finding out about the Job: Job Specifications; Observation of Health Workers; Morbidity and Mortality Data; Community Traditions and Culture; An Analysis of the Health Care System	30
3.4	Writing down the Job as a List of Tasks	34
3.5	How much Detail should be Given?	35
3.6	Conclusion	36

3
Deciding what should be Learnt – an Overview

Perhaps the two most important points made in this book so far are:

(i) Primary Health Care (PHC) is quite different from conventional types of curative care. So when you are thinking about training PHC workers you must start from the beginning rather than copying the kind of training that has been done in the past.
(ii) One of the key roles of a teacher is to decide what the students should learn.

From these starting points this chapter explains the general process of working out what students should learn. This is done in fairly general terms to explain the background. Chapter 4 then goes on to suggest how an individual teacher can apply these general ideas in practice.

3.1 WHAT SHOULD BE THE OVERALL AIM OF A COURSE?

The obvious answer to the question in the heading is 'To help the students learn'.

Whilst this is true, it still leaves the question 'What is the point of this learning?'

One of the assumptions of this book is that:

> Courses should be planned to prepare students for their work in PHC

This is absolutely fundamental. So it will be worth thinking about whether it is correct.

There are many courses where this assumption is not followed. These other courses for health workers are designed to give health workers international qualifications. Or they are designed to give the students as good an understanding as possible of a subject or a discipline—such as Anatomy or Immunology or Parasitology. Sometimes courses are designed to develop the potential of each individual student' or to 'provide an education for life'.

These kinds of overall aims are not themselves bad or harmful. But it is the authors' opinion that these different aims distract from the fundamental purpose of courses in PHC. This purpose is to develop the skills of health workers as far as possible so that the communities which they serve can achieve as high a standard of health as possible. Therefore this chapter starts from our fundamental assumption—that courses should prepare students to do a job.

If this assumption is not accepted, then the whole process of planning courses will be to some extent confused and should not follow the stages outlined below.

(The authors do not feel that *all* courses in all subjects should adopt our assumptions; we are only writing about courses where this assumption is accepted.)

3.2 WHAT ARE THE CONSEQUENCES OF PREPARING STUDENTS TO DO A JOB?

If one accepts that a course should prepare students to do a job, then the course will inevitably reflect this aim. There are four main consequences.

(i) The crucial point about this approach is that

> teachers must know what the job is

This may sound obvious and of course many teachers do know quite well what the job is really like. But there are also a lot of teachers who don't know in any detail what their students will be doing or who don't bother to relate their knowledge of the job very closely to the teaching that they do. For example, teachers sometimes teach their students how to sterilise equipment using an autoclave. In the field, the students will have to work where the nearest autoclave is a hundred miles away so the teaching is not related to the job. Or teachers may spend time telling their health inspector students about 'The Clean Air Act' in Britain or pollution control in the USA when in their own country there is no similar legislation. The time would be better spent in learning how to cast concrete slabs for pit latrines or possibly how to build the slabs from other locally available materials.

(ii) Once the teacher knows exactly what the job is, he or she will be able to decide what to include in the course.

> It is the job itself that determines what will be taught during the course—rather than the teacher's own interests

The basic point is that if something must be learnt in order to do the job well, it should be included in the course. On the other hand, if the thing is not needed for the job, it should be left out.

So, for example, the job of a health worker may involve improving the nutrition of a community by teaching them how to grow beans. So the course must include time for teaching the health worker how to grow the beans—when to plant them, how deeply to plant the seed, etc.,etc. On the other hand, the health worker won't need to know what the Latin name for beans is or which family of plants beans belong to. So these need not be taught.

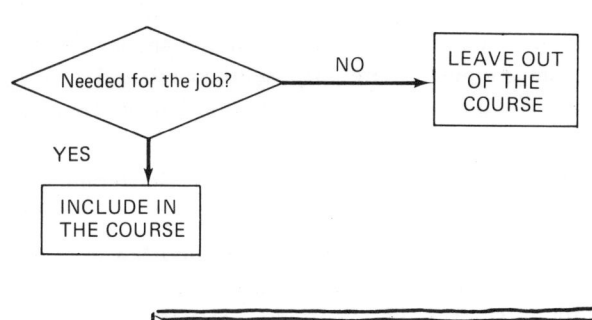

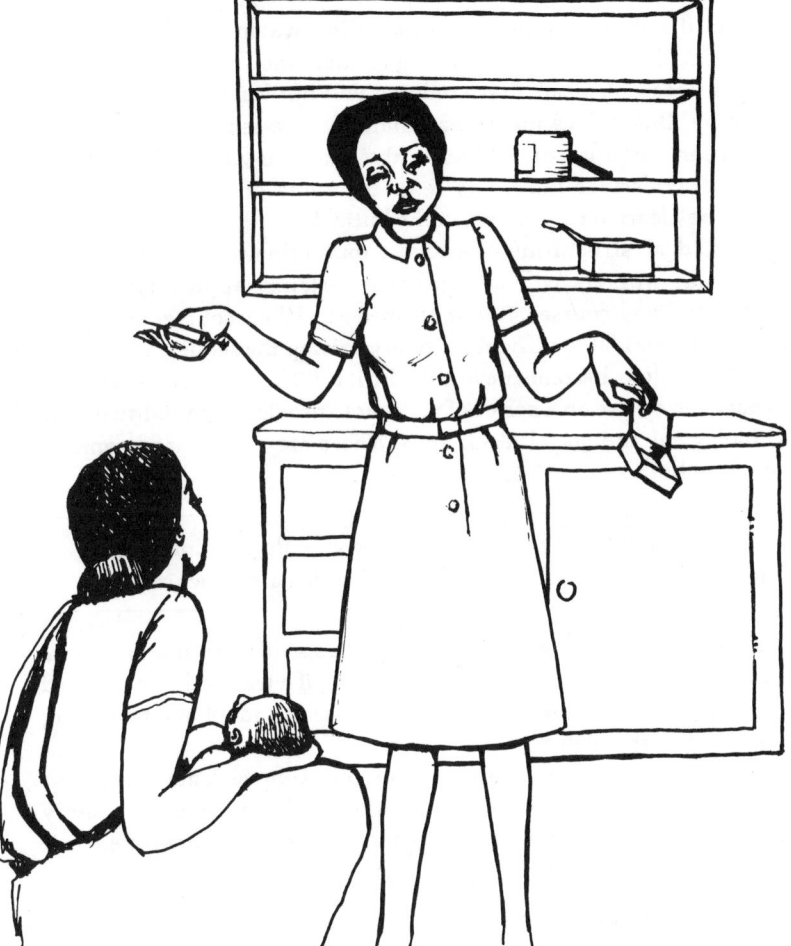

Figure 3.1 There is little point in teaching health workers to use drugs which are not available

As another example, a health worker may have the job of explaining to groups of patients what anaemia is and how it can be reduced by diet, and why it may be necessary to take iron tablets. For this job the students do not need to know the molecular structure of haemoglobin (even though it is very interesting). On the other hand they do need to know various techniques involved in explaining. These techniques are much more than simply telling people the facts. They might include the use of visual aids or using songs or dramas to illustrate the points effectively. So, for this particular job, molecular structure of haemoglobin is 'out'. Use of drama and song is 'in'. The result of all this is a much more purposeful course and it may mean that the course could achieve a similar standard in less time.

(iii) | The structure and sequence of the course will be different

Ideally the teaching should be organised round the work that the health worker will do. This means that the course will not be structured round subjects like anatomy, physiology, nutrition, etc. Instead it will have topics like 'providing water supplies', 'giving intramuscular injections', 'advising on diet', etc.

This does not mean that students will not learn anything about anatomy. But it does mean that anatomy as a separate subject will disappear. The students will learn about anatomy which is needed to give intramuscular injections (e.g. the route of the sciatic nerve) when they learn how to inject in the buttocks.

This 'ideal' structuring of a course round the various tasks which the health workers will do is almost certainly appropriate for all shorter training courses, i.e. up to one year. When courses are longer there are formidable difficulties of organising the sequence of teaching. Repetitions become inevitable. So it is difficult to decide whether to base the course on a series of tasks or to provide an initial structure of biological and social disciplines. There are strong arguments in favour of both alternatives.

(iv) | Teachers on the course will need to be very flexible and ready to teach things which they may not be used to teaching

For example, in the section above it was said that anatomy *as a separate subject* would often disappear. So if a teacher has been used to teaching just anatomy, he or she will need to adapt and be willing to teach different subjects.

Whilst this different approach may mean unwelcome change for some teachers, other teachers may enjoy a new challenge. Certainly it will be helpful to students to have the course more integrated as it will make learning both easier and more purposeful.

We have now explained some of the consequences of this approach. So the next section deals with how teachers or course planners can find out about the job which will be done by the students.

3.3 FINDING OUT ABOUT THE JOB

As explained above, teachers need to know what job the students are going to do. This is not a purely logical step-by-step process which can be explained precisely. In fact it is a little bit confused and information needs to be collected from different sources.

The diagram is intended to show the various sources of information. It is also meant to show that the link between the sources of information and the job is not simple.

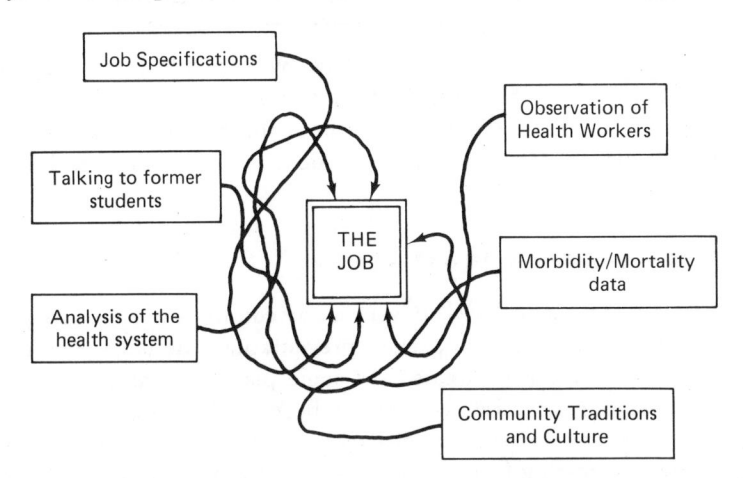

```
    Job Specifications
                              Observation of
                              Health Workers
    Talking to former
    students
                    THE
                    JOB       Morbidity/Mortality
                              data
    Analysis of the
    health system

              Community Traditions
              and Culture
```

The Job Specification

The job specification for a category of health personnel is usually a good starting point. Most Ministries of Health do specify what they expect their health workers to do.

For example in one country, medical assistants are expected to:

(1) Diagnose and treat the more common diseases.
(2) Manage rural health centres.
    etc., etc.

This job specification is a starting point—but it is not enough. Which are the common diseases? What treatments are available? What is meant by manage? Will the medical assistant need to keep financial records? Will he or she be responsible for appointing staff, etc., etc? This kind of job specification does not give the teacher nearly enough detail. But the final description of the job must be consistent with the official job specification.

Observation of Health Workers

This can often fill in a lot of these details and may possibly show that what health workers actually do is rather different from the official intention. For example, in one country nurses are not meant to diagnose. Yet they are often posted to rural areas where they are the only health workers. If they don't diagnose, the patients will have no treatment. So, in practice, the nurses do diagnose and treat patients.

In another country the job specification outlines a very broad range of duties for public health nurses. But what actually happens is that the nurses spend a large proportion of their time administering the distribution of food supplements and so never have time to carry out all the other duties.

> The actual work done may not match the job specification

Teachers and course planners should be aware of this difference. They should decide whether they are going to prepare students for the actual job or the official job—or some combination of these two. (This difference between the 'official' job and the 'actual' job is discussed in more detail in chapter 4.)

Morbidity and Mortality Data

This should also be considered. In very many countries the most frequent causes of death and disablement are preventable. The most commonly occurring diseases can be treated. In some places the health workers' training does not concentrate enough on these conditions and sometimes spends a lot of time on very rare diseases. Of course these rarer diseases may be very interesting from a medical point of view—but that is not the point. The real point is that the health worker should be capable of dealing appropriately with the priorities in health care.

Therefore data about morbidity and mortality should be studied in order to find out what the major health problems are. Then one should make sure that the course will equip the health workers with the appropriate skills.

The Community Traditions and Culture

The community traditions and culture should also be studied as they will almost certainly have an important effect on health. They will also affect how health workers will carry out their work. Examples of the importance of understanding traditions are especially common in the areas of nutrition and child spacing. If a health worker is going to be able to improve the nutrition of a community he or she must understand what the existing diet is—and the reasons for it. For example, there would be little point in encouraging Hindu people to eat beef to give them more protein, as their cattle are sacred.

Community traditions and beliefs can limit the effectiveness of health workers in some places. In others they can be a powerful resource which can help the health worker. Some communities have strong traditions of self-help and working together as a community. Other communities are very compassionate in helping people within the community who are ill, old or disabled.

All these aspects should be learnt by the health worker during the course. But even more important, they should influence the content of the course, so that health workers will be able to provide the services which are important to the community—and provide these services in such a way that they are acceptable to the community.

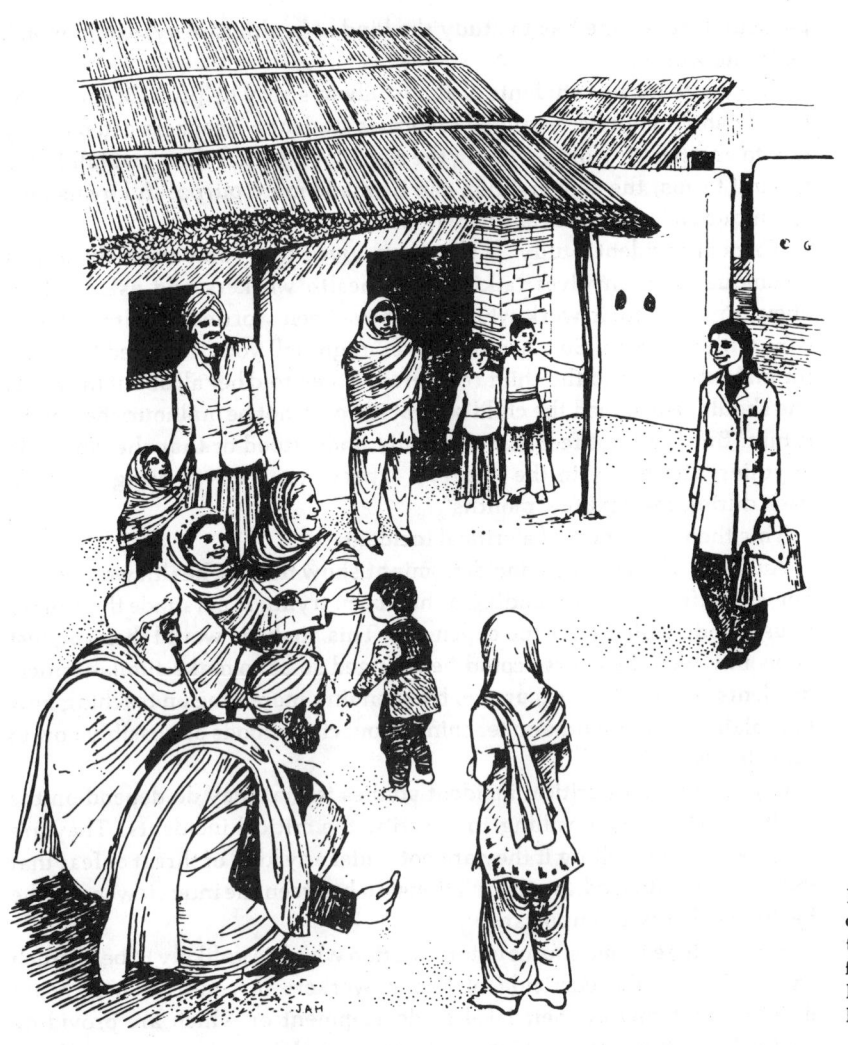

Figure 3.2 Teachers should visit the community to find out about the traditions and culture. (Reproduced from *On Being in Charge*, Rosemary McMahon, Elizabeth Barton and Maurice Piot, WHO, 1980.)

An Analysis of the Health Care System

This is also very important. It should show who the health worker will be working with, what kind of facilities will be available and what kind of work needs to be done.

Suppose that you are planning to train nurses. Your first thought might be that nurses do similar work throughout the world—and so it would be sensible to look at courses in other countries to see how nurses are trained there.

This could be very misleading. What kind of nurse are you training? Will the nurse work in a hospital as a member of a large team? Or, will the nurse be the only health worker in charge of a rural dispensary? Will the nurse be responsible for administering and recording drugs prescribed by a doctor? Or, will she be having to decide what to use when the penicillin has run out? The general title of a 'nurse' does not give nearly enough idea of what the nurse will do—or should do. To understand the job of this particular nurse one has to study the kind of health care system in which he or she works.

Talking to former students is almost always very helpful. Of course the talking should not be restricted to former students. Teachers can usefully talk to any health workers doing the same job. Rather than just talking in general terms, the conversation can be made more purposeful by using a technique called a 'Critical Incident Study'.

'Critical Incident Study' is the name given to a comparatively simple technique. This involves talking with health workers and asking them about times in their work when they have been worried or felt unable to cope with the work. So a health worker might tell you, 'I treated her child for malnutrition and the child recovered. I then told her all about the foods she should use to feed the child so that it would not be malnourished in the future. But I did not feel that she really understood or that she would do anything differently in the future. I expect that she will bring her child back during the next few months'.

This then is a report of a critical incident.

Analysis of this critical incident might show that the health worker was not very effective in persuading or had been trying to persuade the mother to use foods which were too expensive. This analysis would then suggest ways in which the course could be changed so as to make similar critical incidents less likely to occur, i.e. by spending more time on teaching how to explain—or more time on teaching about cheap foods or possibly how to grow foods.

One point about critical incident studies is that they do depend on the health worker being willing to describe the critical incidents. They are only likely to be willing if they are not under any kind of threat or fear that they will be criticised. So the relationship between the interviewer and the health worker is all important.

Finally there is one source of information which is unlikely to be of much value. That is the curricula of health workers in countries which are different in terms of their level of development or which are providing medical/curative care services rather than PHC services. International recognition of qualifications or international standardisation in any form is quite irrelevant to PHC. Primary Health Care is that care which is appropriate in the *local* context and may quite reasonably take a quite different form to health care in neighbouring or distant countries.

3.4 WRITING DOWN THE JOB AS A LIST OF TASKS

The aim of studying all these sources of information is to write down in some detail what the job actually is. The way to do this is to write down the job as a list of tasks.

The tasks will probably be grouped under headings such as:

- Water supplies
- Sanitation
- MCH
- Curative care
- etc., etc.

```
┌─────────────────────────────────────────────────────────┐
│  The job of a ..................................................  │
├─────────────────────────────────────────────────────────┤
│        Tasks                                            │
├─────────────────────────────────────────────────────────┤
│                                                         │
│  1.                                                     │
│                                                         │
└──⌒──────⌒──────⌒──────⌒──────⌒──────⌒──────⌒──────⌒────┘
```

So for example under the heading of water supplies you might put

(i) Preparing a map of a district showing all sources of water.
(ii) Testing water to determine whether it is suitable for drinking.
(iii) Building protection for a spring.
(iv) Encouraging communities to dig wells and showing how to do this.
(v) . . .
(vi) . . . etc., etc.

The essential feature of writing down the tasks is that

> The tasks should be described as things which the health worker does

rather than subjects or topics. For example, the list above makes it reasonably clear that the health worker will be expected to build the protection for springs himself or will actually carry out the testing of water.

If this list had been written as subjects or topics it might have been

distribution of water supplies;
suitability of water for drinking;
protection of springs;
community participation.

These general subjects would not indicate the job to be done, and so would not be helpful in deciding what students should learn.

3.5 HOW MUCH DETAIL SHOULD BE GIVEN?

One problem in writing the tasks is to decide how much detail is needed. The only rule is to provide as much detail as necessary for making decisions about what the students should learn. This rule is fairly obviously sensible, but it is not terribly helpful. An example may illustrate what is needed.

The task might have been written as 'Provide water supplies'. This would not be enough detail. It could mean building a reinforced concrete dam across a river and installing pumping stations and piped supplies. On the other hand it might mean placing some stones round a natural spring.

Both of these very different things could be called 'providing a water supply', so this phrase is not sufficiently detailed.

On the other hand, if the type of water supply is to be a covered well, the task need not specify all the details of exactly what materials will be used for the cover and how they will be placed in position.

> Provide enough detail to specify clearly the nature of the work to be done and the health worker's role in that work

When this stage has been done, you will have a list of tasks which will define the content of the course.

3.6 CONCLUSION

This process of writing down a list of tasks is so important that the next chapter is devoted to explaining in more detail how it can be done in practice by individual teachers.

The importance can be illustrated by the story of the traveller who stopped at a junction to ask, 'Which is the right road?' 'Where do you want to get to?' asked the man at the junction. 'Oh, I don't know', replied the traveller. 'Well, in that case it doesn't matter which road you take.'

Unless travellers know where they are wanting to travel to, they are unlikely to arrive, however fast they travel. In the same way there must be a clear goal when health workers are being trained.

> The goal is that the students will learn all the skills needed in order to provide effective health care

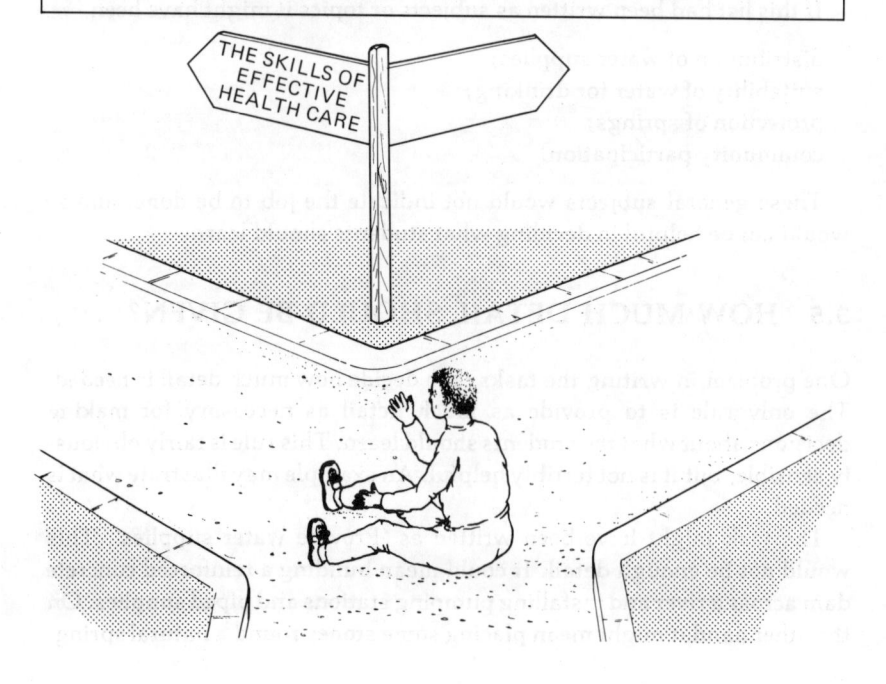

Figure 3.3 The skills of effective health care

SUMMARY

- Courses in PHC should prepare the learners to do their work in PHC.
- To do this, the teacher must know precisely what the job is.
- The teacher can find out about the job by:
    studying job specifications;
    talking to former students;
    studying the community and its traditions;
    observing health workers;
    analysing the health system;
    studying morbidity and mortality data.
- Using this approach will affect the content of the course, the sequence in which it is taught, the teaching methods, and will mean that teachers may have to teach different subjects.

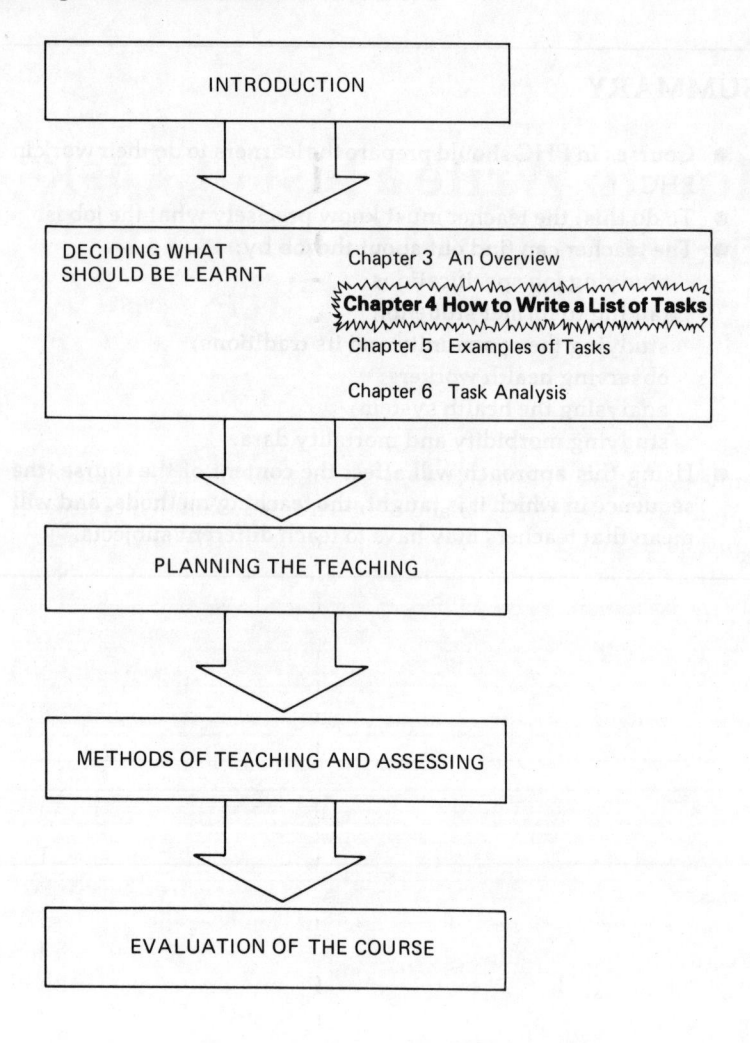

```
        ┌──────────────────┐
        │   INTRODUCTION   │
        └──────────────────┘
                 ↓
        ┌──────────────────────────────────────────────┐
        │ DECIDING WHAT      Chapter 3  An Overview    │
        │ SHOULD BE LEARNT   ≈≈Chapter 4 How to Write a List of Tasks≈≈
        │                    Chapter 5  Examples of Tasks │
        │                    Chapter 6  Task Analysis  │
        └──────────────────────────────────────────────┘
                 ↓
        ┌──────────────────────┐
        │ PLANNING THE TEACHING│
        └──────────────────────┘
                 ↓
        ┌────────────────────────────────────┐
        │ METHODS OF TEACHING AND ASSESSING  │
        └────────────────────────────────────┘
                 ↓
        ┌──────────────────────────┐
        │ EVALUATION OF THE COURSE │
        └──────────────────────────┘
```

CONTENTS

4.1	Making the Draft List of Tasks for your Course	39
4.2	Improving the Task List by Considering Curricula, Job Descriptions and Manuals	42
4.3	Improving the Task List by Comparing it with the Health Needs of the Community	45
4.4	Improving the Task List by Observing a Health Worker at Work	47
4.5	Conclusion	48

4
How to Write a List of Tasks for a Training Course in Primary Health Care

Chapter 3 explained that deciding what students should learn can be done by finding out about the job and then writing down a list of tasks. This chapter is a 'how to' chapter. It explains in detail how a teacher can prepare a list of tasks which he will teach.

There are four stages suggested in writing a list of tasks. These are:

(1) Writing a draft list of tasks by thinking about the work which will be done by the students after they have completed their training.
(2) Improving the list by considering curricula and job specifications.
(3) Improving the list by comparing it with community health needs and local cultures.
(4) Improving the list by observing health workers and talking to them.

At the end of this process each course will have a list of tasks. The list should be unique for each course. This is because each category of health workers performs different jobs in different countries. So, although some tasks will appear on almost all lists of tasks, each course will have a different balance and different details reflecting the unique health problems, cultures and health systems of the individual situations.

> The list of tasks will be different for each training course and for each country

The following section explains how each stage can be done.

4.1 MAKING THE DRAFT LIST OF TASKS FOR YOUR COURSE

Start by trying to *forget* the classroom, the textbook, the examination questions and the way you have been teaching in the past.

Start with a fresh mind and a blank piece of paper.

(i) Now think about your students after they have left you and have started working in the community. Imagine all those things you would like your students to do well at the end of the course. Think about all the aspects of the work they will do and then write it down.

> *For example*, you might write that you would like them to:
> - introduce themselves politely to the leaders and people of the community;
> - get to know the people and understand their beliefs;
> - find out the main problems affecting people's health.

Sometimes important tasks such as these are not written down in the curriculum or in the job description. They are assumed to be 'common sense' or are regarded as obvious. But experience shows that health workers often do not understand their community. So these 'common sense' tasks need to be learnt. If they are not learnt, the health workers will be much less effective. This is because good relationships with the people and the community are the foundation of successful health care.

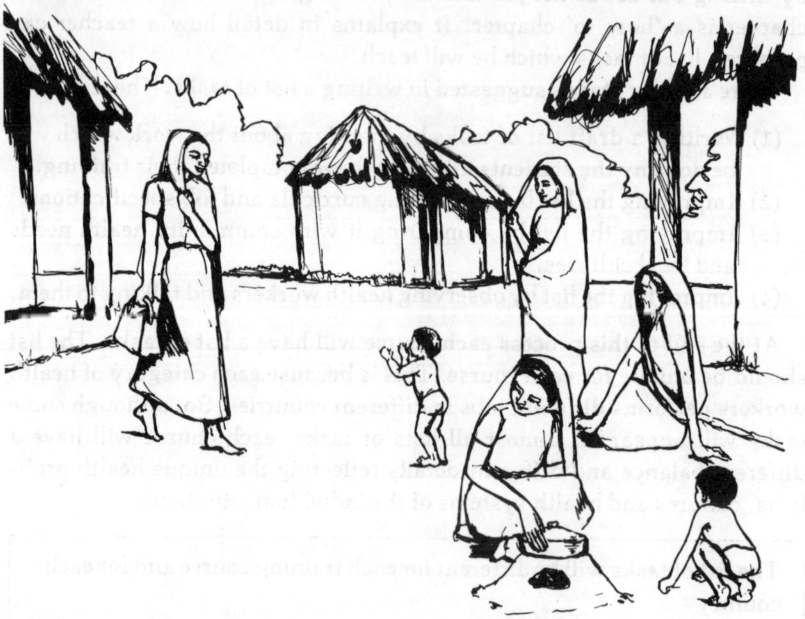

Figure 4.1 The list of tasks should include tasks such as 'Getting to know the people in the community'

(ii) Now, keep on imagining the daily life of your student when he starts work.

> *For example*, what happens when he goes to work in the morning? You might write that you would expect him or her:
> - to supervise that the building where he works is kept clean and the surrounding environment is free of rubbish;
> - to maintain a pit latrine at the health centre as a model—free of flies and mosquitoes and with clean surroundings;
> - keep the drugs and other stocks well labelled and in good order.

(iii) Now imagine your student's work and think of the various parts of his job. Is he always in one place? Or does he travel between villages? Does he or she go home-visiting or conduct clinics at different places? Is there a need to plan these various activities?

> *For example*, you might write that you would expect your student to:
> - make a weekly timetable for himself and the other members of the health care team;
> - make a duty roster for the health centre staff.

It is sometimes important for health workers to learn how to use *time*. This is especially important when a health worker has several aspects of his work such as clinics, home-visiting, health education and work in surrounding villages. The greater the variety of the work, the more important it is for him to learn how to plan his time.

(iv) Now, there are also technical parts of his job. By this we mean the skills of being a midwife or a sanitarian or a nutritionist. These will make a very long list—and these are the aspects most commonly included in a curriculum or a job description. But you will find that when you rewrite the curriculum in the form of tasks, the list will be of practical value for planning the teaching.

> *For example*, if the curriculum says 'Conduct an antenatal clinic' then the performances for an antenatal clinic in the village might be:
> - take an obstetric history from a pregnant woman and fill in the details on the antenatal card;
> - clinically examine a pregnant woman to detect
>   —anaemia
>   —pre-eclamptic toxaemia
>   —abnormalities in lie and presentation
>   and refer or treat as appropriate;
> - decide which patients are at risk and when to refer them;
> - and so on.

(v) Now, still continue imagining your student with his daily work. Perhaps he comes across a problem and he does not know what to do. It is something he has not been taught to manage.

> *For example*, you might write that you would like your student to:
> - recognise conditions that he cannot manage and refer to the hospital;
> - refer problems connected with water supplies to the District Water Authority;
> - or arrange transport for an obstetric emergency to be taken to hospital.

(vi) Now you might like to check with chapter 5. This gives a list of examples of the tasks which various types of health care worker might do.

Use these lists to help you think of more things which your students will do when they are health workers in the field.

Summary

At this point you have a long list of all the tasks you would like your students to do well when they start work.

These tasks should all specify the action, communication or decision that the health worker will perform. This is, they should emphasise fairly precisely what the health worker will *do*.

4.2 IMPROVING THE DRAFT LIST OF TASKS BY CONSIDERING CURRICULA, JOB DESCRIPTIONS AND MANUALS

> At the end of this section you will be able to answer the question 'Do the tasks include all of the tasks implied in the job description, curricula and manuals?'

The task list you have written will contain most of the performances your student will do in his job. But to make it more complete and more practical it needs to be modified by comparing it with what other people have thought. Their ideas may have been written down as a curriculum for the training course, as a job specification or possibly as a manual.

It is important to consider and include these other ideas, as well as your own. It would obviously be wrong to only take into account your own ideas because the health workers will probably have to work for a Ministry of Health. So the training programme must fit their ideas.

One problem is that the curriculum, manual or job description may not be written as a list of tasks. (Ideally all of these documents should be very clear about which tasks need to be performed; in practice this often does not happen.)

Common problems with these documents include:

They may be written in vague language.

For example, 'he will treat common conditions'. This does not say *which* common conditions or *what* he will do to treat them.

They may be written in broad general terms.

For example, 'he will detect specific hazards in the community which lead to disease'. This does not say which hazards or how they will be detected.

They may be written in words which state goals but not the activities (tasks) which achieve those goals.

For example, 'he will improve the nutritional status of children under five years'. But what tasks are needed to achieve this?

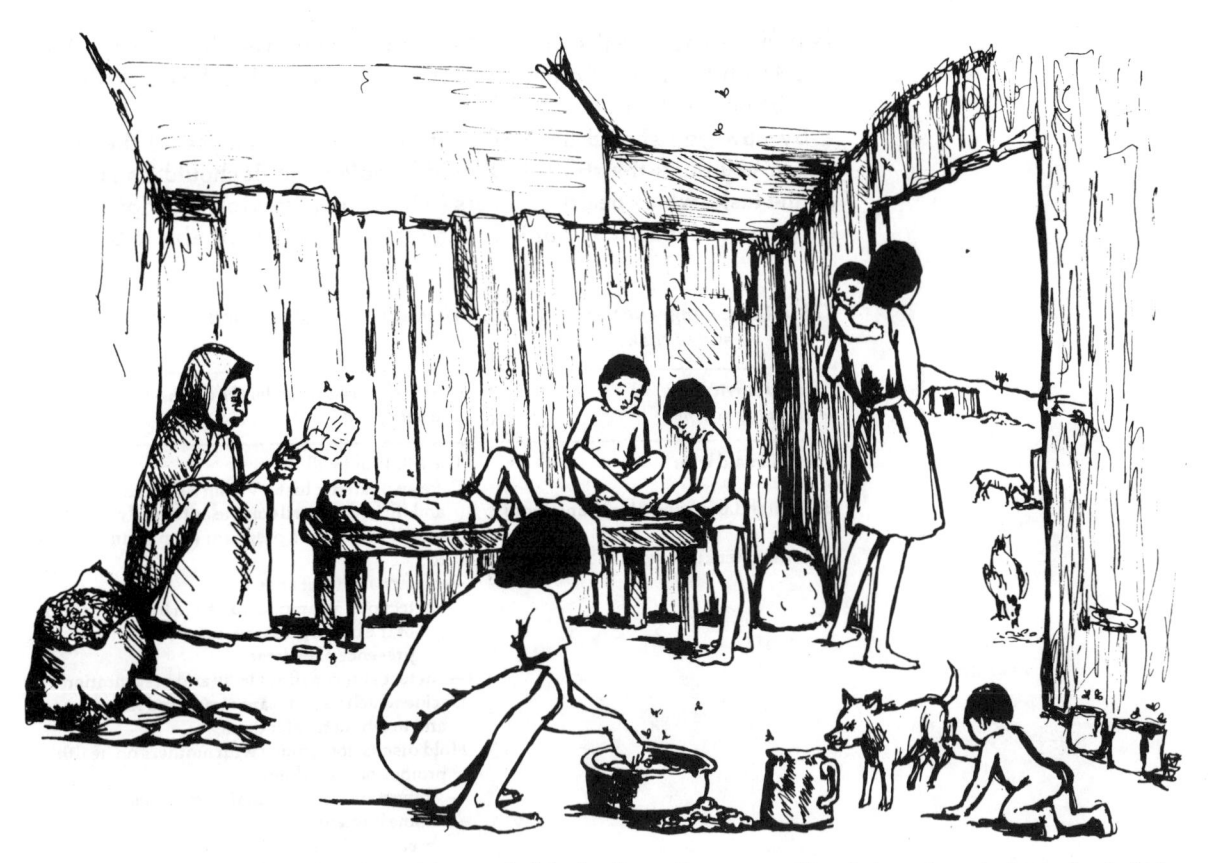

Figure 4.2 'He will detect hazards in the community which lead to disease' is too vague. How the hazards can be detected and which hazards to look for should be stated

Now study the curriculum, the job description or manuals. Then, improve the task list you have written by adding those things mentioned in the curriculum which you have forgotten. Change the wording used in the curriculum into wording which states a task. See some examples of how to do this in table 4.1. If there are things in the curriculum which you cannot state as tasks, put these in a separate list and head it 'enabling factors' (see chapter 6).

Now compare your original list of tasks with the list of tasks given in the curriculum or in the job specification. There might be items on your draft list which are not mentioned in the curriculum. For example, 'supervise the cleaning of the health centre' or 'understand the people's customs'.

Should a teacher remove items from his list if they are not mentioned in the curriculum or job specification?

The answer is:

NO (do not remove from your list)
— if the tasks help in the performance of the main job;
— if the tasks are within the scope and spirit of the training programme.

YES (remove from your list)
— if the teacher's tasks are seriously inconsistent with the job specification or curriculum;

— if the teacher's tasks would take too much time to teach (i.e. they would prevent teaching of other important tasks implied in the curriculum or job specification).

By now you should have a list of tasks which includes all the things which you think the students should be able to do. It should also include all the tasks which health planners (who have written job descriptions and curricula and manuals) think that the students should be able to do.

Table 4.1 Change the wording of a curriculum or job description into a list of stated tasks

Part of a curriculum as given to a teacher	Curriculum rewritten by the teacher as a list of tasks
The MCH aid will: Understand the principles of antenatal care Perform antenatal care in the village	The MCH aid will: Take an obstetric history from a pregnant woman and fill in the details on the antenatal card Clinically examine a pregnant woman and be able to: — detect and treat anaemia — detect pre-eclamptic toxaemia by examination of the blood pressure, urine protein and presence of oedema — detect abnormalities in lie and presentation Decide which patients are at risk and know when and to whom to refer them Hold discussion groups with mothers on health promotion including: — importance of antenatal attendance — home hygiene — breast feeding — weaning foods — nutrition during pregnancy and lactation

Part of a job description as given to a teacher	Job description written as list of tasks
The health worker will: Improve the nutritional status of children	The health worker will: Assess the nutritional status of children under 5 years by: weight-age graphs and mid-arm circumference measurements Promote the importance of breast feeding Devise weaning foods based on locally grown products Train mothers in the preparation of weaning foods to supplement breast feeding Teach mothers how to prevent diarrhoea in young children and train them in early treatment with oral rehydration fluids and so on

4.3 IMPROVING THE TASK LIST BY COMPARING IT WITH THE HEALTH NEEDS OF THE COMMUNITY

> At the end of this step you should be able to answer the question 'Do the tasks you have listed relate to important and specific health needs of the community?'

Your list so far includes your ideas as a teacher and the ideas of planners as they have expressed them in curricula and job specifications. These ideas should already have taken into account community health needs and the local culture and traditions. However this is not always the case. So you should make a point now of specifically thinking about the list of tasks from the point of view of the community.

The overall pattern you should follow is to first identify the health problems and resources in the community. Then you should work out what the health worker will need to do in order to respond to these needs and resources. Finally you should compare this new list of tasks with the list you already have and make the necessary changes. The way that you can do this is set out below.

Find out as much as you reasonably can about the health needs of the community, and the resources within the community. Do this by:

- Looking at any morbidity/mortality data which is available. (Be careful here, because often this data is based only on what happens at health centres and hospitals. So there may be a lot of unreported illness.)
- Talking to people in the community to find out what they think the main health problems are. Find out also how they deal with illness within the community (e.g. what do they do when a small child has diarrhoea), how they get water, what food they eat.

What are the important health needs of the community where your students will work? Which of those needs will be the responsibility of your students?

The health needs of a community need to be stated specifically. For example:

- some places need new wells;
- others have wells but the pumps need maintenance;
- other places need to get water by pipes from protected springs.

It is not sufficient to say 'help community water supply'. The specific task which will help the community needs must be stated.

Now ask the following questions.

- Are there important needs which are not met by the tasks on your list? (Add appropriate tasks which will meet the community need.)
- Are there items on your task list which do not seem important in this community (mark these and give them low priority in your teaching course).

The health needs of most communities cover such a wide range that to list them would fill a book! It is not possible for one health worker to fulfil all these needs. Usually there are several categories of health worker in an area, with different functions. But often these functions overlap. In this case, areas of main responsibility and secondary responsibility should be understood and defined. (See example in table 4.2.)

Table 4.2 *Some health-promoting activities needed by a community*

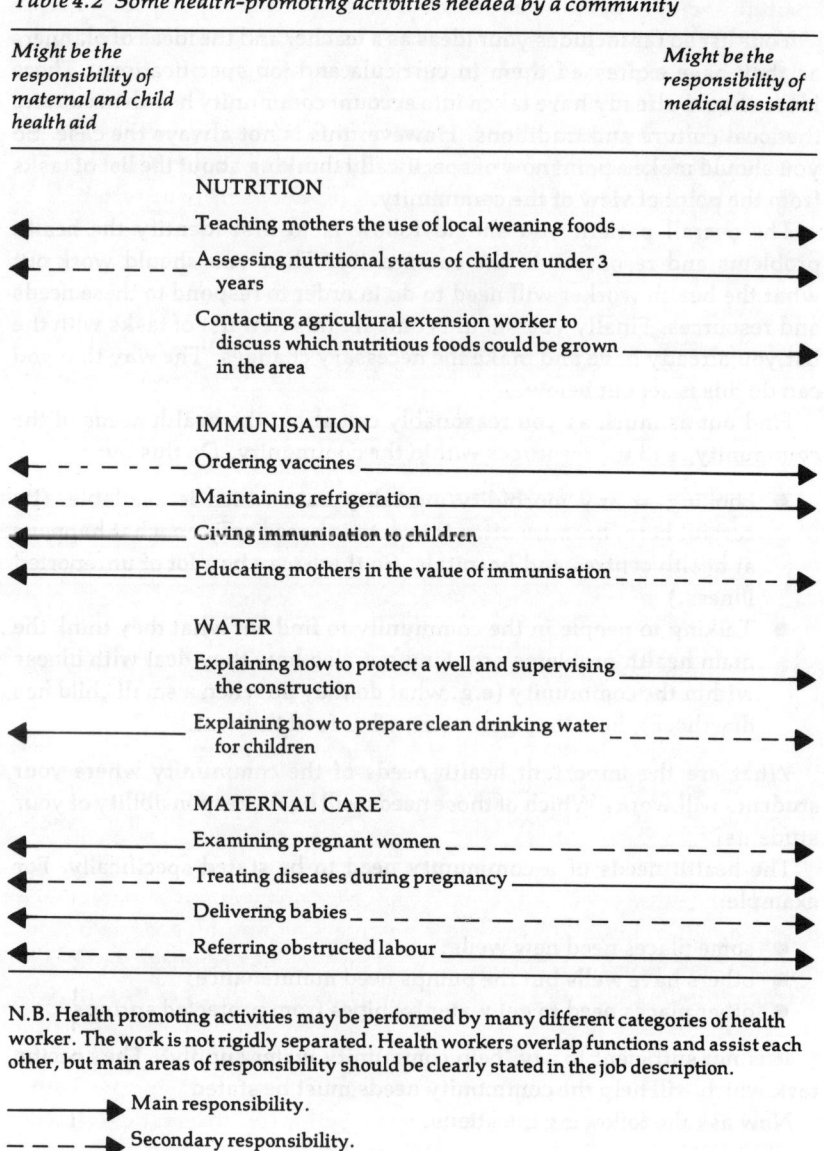

Might be the responsibility of maternal and child health aid		Might be the responsibility of medical assistant
	NUTRITION	
←——————	Teaching mothers the use of local weaning foods	——————→
←——————	Assessing nutritional status of children under 3 years	
	Contacting agricultural extension worker to discuss which nutritious foods could be grown in the area	——————→
	IMMUNISATION	
←——————	Ordering vaccines	
←——————	Maintaining refrigeration	
←——————	Giving immunisation to children	
←——————	Educating mothers in the value of immunisation	——————→
	WATER	
	Explaining how to protect a well and supervising the construction	——————→
←——————	Explaining how to prepare clean drinking water for children	——————→
	MATERNAL CARE	
←——————	Examining pregnant women	——————→
←——————	Treating diseases during pregnancy	
←——————	Delivering babies	——————→
←——————	Referring obstructed labour	

N.B. Health promoting activities may be performed by many different categories of health worker. The work is not rigidly separated. Health workers overlap functions and assist each other, but main areas of responsibility should be clearly stated in the job description.

——————▶ Main responsibility.

— — —▶ Secondary responsibility.

4.4 IMPROVING THE TASK LIST BY OBSERVING A HEALTH WORKER AT WORK

> At the end of this step you should be able to answer the question: 'are these tasks practised in the community situation?'

There may be health workers previously trained by your school or institute and now working in the community, or there may be other health workers trained previously on other courses but doing similar work.

It is very useful for a teacher to visit these workers.

The purpose is to find out:
- what are the practical difficulties he faces in his daily work?
- what are the common problems which people bring to him?
- which part of his training is he using (or not using) and why?

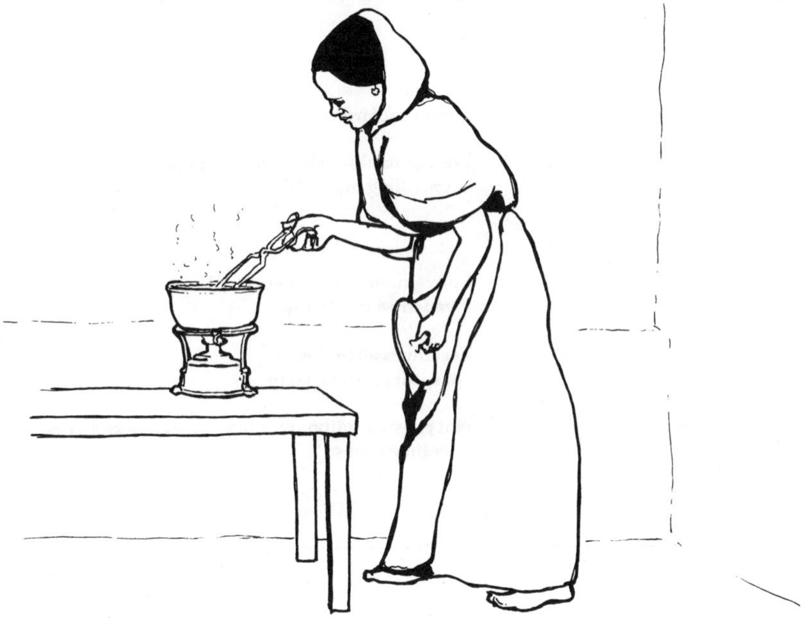

Figure 4.3 A syllabus may include sterilisation using an autoclave—but the health worker in the field may have to use a pan of boiling water

Visit a health worker and spend as much time as you can (a whole day if possible) observing him/her. Write down everything he does as a task. Always include things not directly related to his technical work. For example, finding out why the cleaner did not come that day or writing a letter to headquarters about his drug shortages. He will probably perform better because you are watching but the problems he faces will be the same.

Hold discussion with him *after* your period of observation. If you discuss too much before you will influence his behaviour. Try to find out:
- why there are things he does not do;
- what are his greatest difficulties;
- which parts of his training helped him;
- which parts of his training are not being used.

Table 4.3 Example of a task list made from observations of and discussions with a maternity aid conducting an antenatal clinic

List of performances expected	Frequency of performance	Comment
Encourages pregnant women to attend antenatal clinic regularly by explaining its importance and use	R	Has not been taught how to do this during training—has only been taught that it must be done!
Selects 'at risk' maternity cases from a study of the obstetric history	N	Has not been taught the 'at risk' method of selective care
Determines the lie, position and presentation of the foetus by palpation of the pregnant abdomen	F	Was taught in initial training
Recognises abnormalities of lie and presentation	F	Has been well trained in this
Predicts difficult deliveries following palpation, and refers such patients for hospital delivery	S	Patients do not always agree. Often no transport available
Examines women clinically and recognises clinical anaemia	F	
Gives out iron tablets to pregnant women	S	Shortage of iron tablets
Refers women with severe anaemia in the last trimester of pregnancy for blood transfusion	R	Women unable to leave their family. Relatives often unwilling to give blood
Examines feet of pregnant women for oedema	F	
Examines blood pressure	N	Sphygmomanometer sent to District Hospital for repairs 6 months ago
Examines urine for protein	N	Test tubes all broken. No spirit for spirit lamp
Diagnoses pre-eclamptic toxaemia	N	Not possible without the blood pressure and urine examinations
and so on		

N, never; S, sometimes; R, rarely; F, frequently.

4.5 CONCLUSION

Now you should have a task list which:

- expresses the intentions of the curriculum and includes all the skills needed for the job;
- deals with the most important community needs within the scope of your students' job function;
- is practical, feasible and relevant within the working situation.

How can this list be used in teaching?

In chapter 5 we give examples of tasks within the different elements of Primary Health Care.

In chapter 6 we discuss how to analyse tasks and how to use this in selecting the teaching method.

In chapter 7 we discuss how to group tasks into a planned teaching programme.

In chapters 10–14 we discuss how to teach and assess the various skills needed to perform the tasks well.

> The overall importance of this task list is that it determines exactly what will be taught—and what will be left out of the course

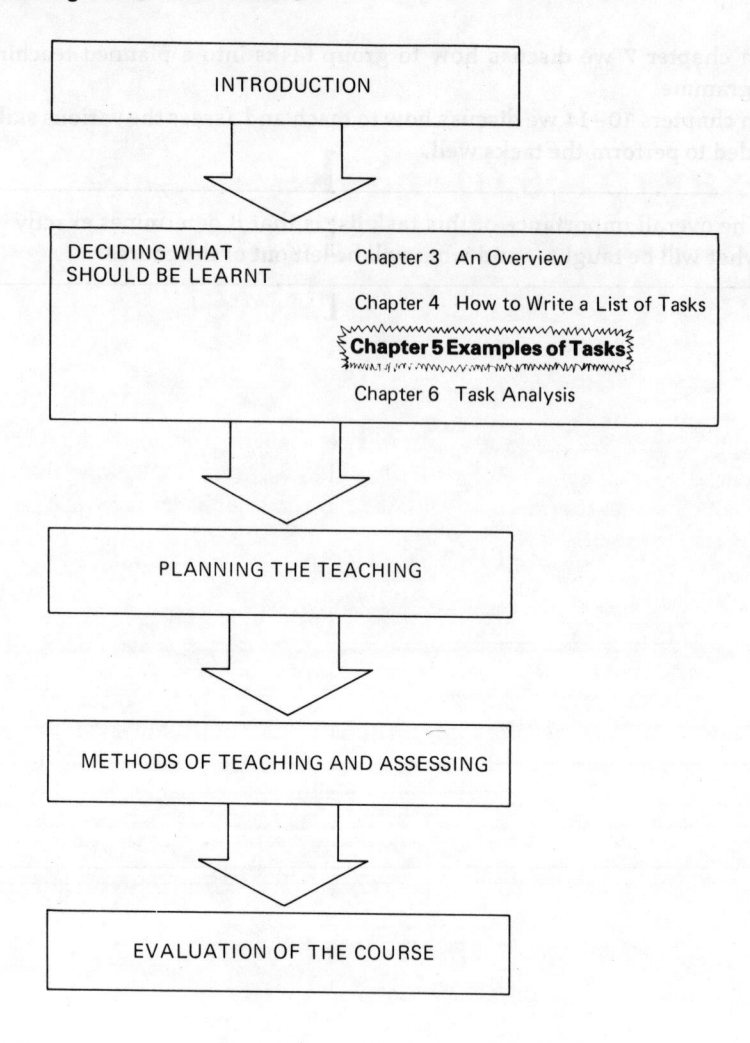

```
         ┌──────────────────┐
         │   INTRODUCTION   │
         └────────┬─────────┘
                  ▼
┌─────────────────────────────────────────────┐
│ DECIDING WHAT        Chapter 3  An Overview │
│ SHOULD BE LEARNT                            │
│                      Chapter 4  How to Write a List of Tasks │
│                      ~~~~~~~~~~~~~~~~~~~~~~~~~~~~~~~~~~~~~~ │
│                      Chapter 5 Examples of Tasks │
│                      ~~~~~~~~~~~~~~~~~~~~~~~~~~~~~~~~~~~~~~ │
│                      Chapter 6  Task Analysis │
└─────────────────────┬───────────────────────┘
                      ▼
         ┌────────────────────────┐
         │   PLANNING THE TEACHING │
         └────────────┬───────────┘
                      ▼
      ┌────────────────────────────────┐
      │ METHODS OF TEACHING AND ASSESSING │
      └────────────────┬───────────────┘
                       ▼
         ┌────────────────────────┐
         │ EVALUATION OF THE COURSE │
         └────────────────────────┘
```

CONTENTS

5.1	Who Performs PHC Tasks?	51
5.2	The Tasks of the PHC Worker: Administrative Tasks; Technical Tasks	51
5.3	The Problem-solving Process	54
5.4	A Classification of Problem-solving Tasks	55
5.5	Examples of Tasks Related to the PHC Elements: Immunisation; Nutrition; Maternal Care; Water; Sanitation; Health Education; Treatment	55

5
Examples of Tasks Performed by Primary Health Care Workers

In this chapter we give a few examples of General Tasks which might be undertaken by Primary Health Care (PHC) workers. By looking through these tasks a teacher may be reminded of some aspect of the work he has forgotten to include in his task list.

5.1 WHO PERFORMS PRIMARY HEALTH CARE TASKS?

As explained in chapter 1 PHC is different from curative hospital care and one of the main differences concerns who performs the tasks. In PHC, the tasks which promote health are performed by family members in the home and by the community in the village, as well as by the health workers (see table 1.1 in chapter 1). It follows from this that a central activity of the PHC worker is Health Education. The central task of the PHC worker is

> To advise and encourage the family and community
> To undertake those tasks which promote health

A PHC worker may be working in one or more of the elements of PHC (Nutrition, Water, Sanitation, Maternal Care and so on). But which ever element he works in, the central and basic tasks will be related to health education. This is why health education is the centre of our PHC Circle (figure 5.1). We have reproduced this diagram here for use when referring to the examples of tasks.

In our lists of tasks we have included only those tasks performed by PHC workers—but it must be remembered that in PHC tasks are also performed by the family and the community. Although these family and community tasks are not included in our lists, the fundamental work of health education to encourage the people to undertake health-promoting tasks applies to every list and to every element of PHC.

5.2 THE TASKS OF THE PHC WORKER

It is convenient to group the tasks of the PHC worker into two main areas: these may be called (i) Administrative tasks, (ii) Technical tasks.

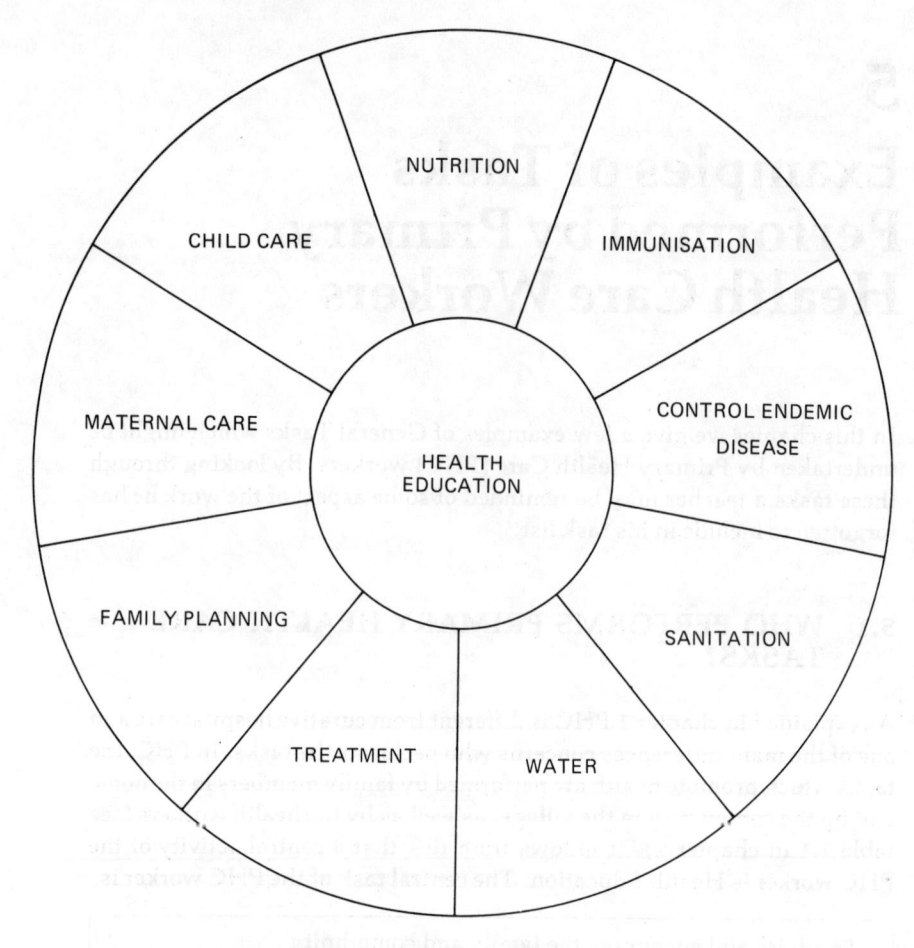

Figure 5.1 The Circle of Primary Health Care

(i) Administrative Tasks

These tasks concern the maintenance of the working environment in which health work is carried out. Maintaining a working environment includes the following general tasks:

- liaising with the District Medical Officer and other officials who are responsible for the supplies and supervision of the health facility;
- ordering and storing supplies and equipment;
- maintaining buildings and supervising repairs;
- keeping registers and preparing reports;
- supervising colleagues;
- working with the village health committee.

These kinds of tasks are often forgotten in the design of curricula but they are an essential aspect of work in many PHC situations. A good PHC teacher will include training in these tasks. (Some detailed examples of this kind of task have been given in chapter 4, section 4.1 (ii) and (iii).)

(ii) Technical Tasks

These are tasks which concern the actual health work of the PHC worker. We have listed some general tasks under headings which indicate the element (or area) of the PHC work. In some cases, for convenience, we have divided the tasks into those related to Community Health Care and those related to Individual Patient Care.

But writing down a heading of an area or element of work is not enough to indicate what the health worker actually does. If the heading for example is Water, what does he do about water? What is done in the health field, and particularly what is done in PHC is almost always a *problem-solving activity*. And so we have looked at the problem-solving activities of each element, to help us list the tasks.

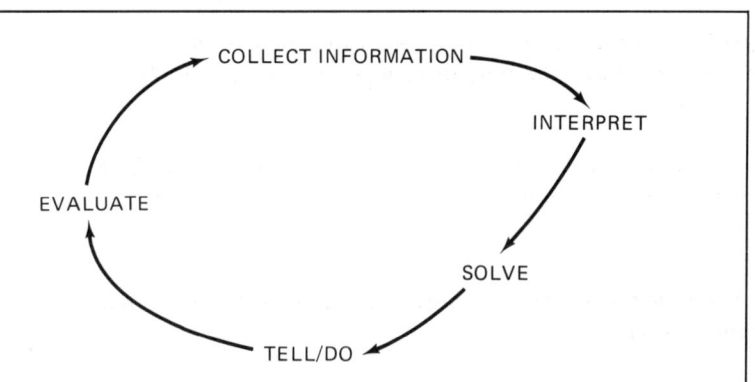

```
        COLLECT INFORMATION
                              ↘
                              INTERPRET
                                ↓
  EVALUATE                    SOLVE
         ↖                  ↙
             TELL/DO
```

The diagram above shows the stages in a simple problem-solving process.

```
        Collect information
                              ↘
                              Interpret
                                ↓
  Evaluate                    solve
         ↖                  ↙
             tell/do
```

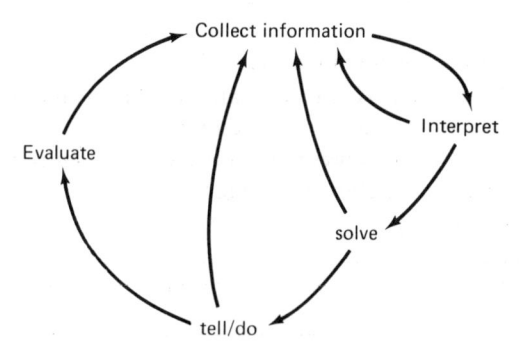

This diagram shows that real problem-solving is more complicated. This is because as we proceed through a problem solving process it is often found that more information is needed before solving a problem.
Sometimes after an activity has begun difficulties arise which need more information before they can be overcome.
In practice problem solving in real life is even more complicated than this.

5.3 THE PROBLEM-SOLVING PROCESS

The problem-solving process has a common pattern. It goes through several stages which are classified below in a simple form. Solving problems is not always as straightforward and linear as these stages imply. Above are shown two diagrams which indicate some of the sidelines which may need to be taken to solve problems. But for the purpose of listing a few examples of general tasks we have used the straight line classification, as shown below.

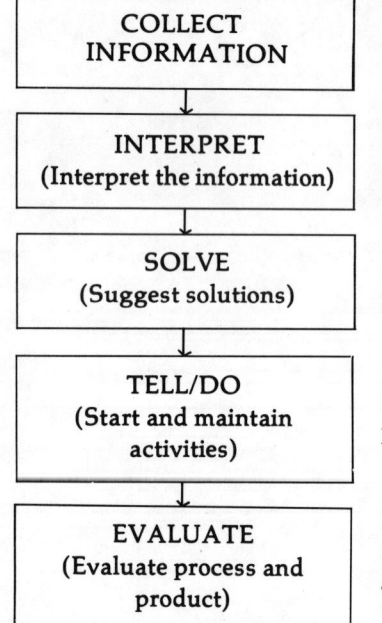

COLLECT INFORMATION (look at the people, the customs, the health problems)

↓

INTERPRET (Interpret the information) (what are the main dangers, what are the causes of the problems, what is the diagnosis, what are the priorities?)

↓

SOLVE (Suggest solutions) (suggest ways and means to solve the problems, action plans, projects or programmes)

↓

TELL/DO (Start and maintain activities) (explain to the community, organise action, perform technical procedures)

↓

EVALUATE (Evaluate process and product) (collect data and make judgements about whether the activities are proceeding well? Is the situation improving?)

Examples of the tasks are now given as tables.
The columns refer to the PHC element, and to whether the activity relates more to the community or more to the patient.
The rows refer to the main stages of the problem-solving process.
The outline of each table is shown in table 5.1.

Table 5.1 The PHC element

Problem-solving process	Tasks with the community	Tasks with the patient
Collect information		
Interpret information		
Suggest or decide on solution		
Start and maintain activities		
Evaluate process and product		

5.4 A CLASSIFICATION OF PROBLEM-SOLVING TASKS RELATED TO PHC ELEMENTS (TABLE 5.2)

Table 5.2

Problem-solving process	Tasks in community	Seeing the patient
Collect information	What is the situation with reference to the particular PHC element?	Take the history Examine the patient Investigate the patient
Interpret information	What are the possible causes of existing problems? Which are priority areas? What are the hazards?	Make a provisional diagnosis

Suggest or decide on solutions	What are the possible
	   actions,
	   training
	   education
	which might improve things
	Decide to take a certain action
		Outline patient-management plan

Start and maintain activities	Explain the problem to the community Organise community action Perform the technical activity	Explain the management to the patient Give the treatment
Evaluate process and product	Are the activities well done? Is the situation improving?	Has the treatment been completed? Has the patient's condition improved?

5.5 EXAMPLES OF TASKS RELATED TO THE PHC ELEMENTS

Tables 5.3 to 5.11 give a few examples of tasks which may be carried out by PHC workers. *They are not a complete list of all possible tasks.*

The reason for including these examples is to illustrate what is meant by the headings 'collect information' or 'evaluate'. The examples may also help to stimulate ideas about all the other tasks which PHC workers do.

Table 5.3 Tasks related to immunisation of the children in the community

Collect information	Assess the level of immunisation of children in the community by
	   —doing a tally of clinic records
	   —estimating the percentage of clinic attenders

Interpret information	Find out, by discussion, the reasons for a low immunisation status, such as
	   community is not aware of the service
	   community does not think immunisation is important
	   immunisation clinics are irregular

(Continued overleaf)

Table 5.3 Tasks related to immunisation of the children in the community (contd)

Suggest solutions	The community should know more about the value of immunisation The regularity of the vaccine supply should be improved
Start and maintain activities	Maintain a refrigerator Order and keep an adequate supply of vaccines Organise regular visits to outlying areas Encourage mothers in regular clinic attendance
Evaluate	Assess children's immunisation status every few years Find out whether the proportion of children who are immunised has changed

Table 5.4 Tasks related to immunisation of individual children

Collect information	Examine the health card and find out which immunisations the child has received Examine the general condition of the child Detect any contraindications to immunisation
Interpret information	Interpret the evidence—which may be conflicting—and decide what age the child is and what immunisations have been received From the age of the child, previous immunisations and condition, decide which immunisations are needed
Suggest solutions	Write out the dates and times of future immunisations based on the national schedule
Start and maintain activities	Explain to the mother the value of immunisation Explain to the mother when to bring the child for the whole course of immunisation Give immunisations for the six diseases of childhood (TB, Polio, Diphtheria, Tetanus, Whooping Cough and Measles)
Evaluate	Check the child's card regularly until immunisation is complete

Table 5.5 Tasks related to nutrition in the community

Collect information	Find out in detail a community's food customs and taboos List locally available foods, their seasonality and availability Assess the prevalence and types of malnutrition in the community Assess the factors associated with malnutrition Discuss with the community what they feel should be done to improve nutrition
Interpret information	Identify the groups most seriously affected by malnutrition Identify the factors of most significance in causing malnutrition (alcohol, poverty, cash crops, inefficient agriculture, ignorance, hungry season, and so on)
Suggest solutions	Prepare a plan of activities directed towards improving the factors of major significance (as identified above)

Table 5.5 Tasks related to nutrition in the community (contd)

Start and maintain activities	Seek the agreement of the community to implement the plan
Encourage the community to grow more protein-containing foods (e.g. beans, pulses)
Encourage mothers to plant vegetable gardens
Educate mothers in correct child feeding
Contact agricultural department to improve local food supplies
Evaluate	Assess increases in community food production
Assess changes in family food consumption

Table 5.6 Tasks related to nutrition in individual children

Collect information	Assess growth in children by
weighing and making age–weight graphs
measuring mid-arm circumference
Take a nutrition history from the mother
Examine a child for signs of malnutrition and associated conditions
Interpret information	Diagnose the different types of malnutrition (anaemia, protein-calorie malnutrition, vitamin deficiencies)
Identify the dietary deficiencies which have created the problem
Identify associated conditions (e.g. helminthic infestation)
Suggest solutions	Outline a plan for the dietary management of the malnourished child
Outline a plan for associated medical treatments (antihelminthic, iron tablets and so on)
Start and maintain activities	Explain to mothers the values of breast feeding, correct weaning foods and frequent feeding of young children
Demonstrate preparation of weaning foods
Treat the child
Establish a long-term follow-up system
Evaluate	Assess the child's growth curve at intervals

Table 5.7 Tasks related to maternal care (antenatal patients only)

Collect information	Take obstetric history from women
Examine the antenatal mother to detect
—anaemia
—pre-eclamptic toxaemia
—abnormalities of foetus or foetal position
—other illness
Interpret information	Decide the EDD (Expected Date of Delivery)
Decide whether the mother's condition is normal or abnormal
Decide whether the mother will be at-risk during delivery
Suggest solutions	Prescribe treatment for detected conditions
Refer the patient when necessary
Decide where labour should take place
Start and maintain activities	Explain to mother how to care for her health and nutrition during pregnancy
Give anti-tetanus immunisation
Give anti-anaemia treatment
Treat the common conditions of pregnancy
Evaluate	Assess whether mother's condition is fit for delivery

Table 5.8 Tasks related to water in a rural community

Collect information	Investigate the sources from which the community draws its water
	Examine each source and determine: its adequacy, its degree of contamination and the methods by which it is collected
	Estimate the seriousness/frequency of water-borne diseases within a community
Interpret information	Define the 'water problem' of this community, is it —inadequate quantities of water —seasonal shortages of water —distance of the collecting points —contamination at source —contamination within the household?
Suggest solutions	Suggest methods of increasing water quantities
	Suggest methods of protecting water sources from contamination
Start and maintain activities	Explain to the people the health hazards related to water
	Protect the following types of water supply: well, spring, dam, river
	Collect and transmit water by gravity flow
	Assemble and install a pump in a well
	Advise villagers on local methods to reduce contamination
Evaluate	Assess the household quantity of water
	Estimate the level of water contamination
	Estimate the level of water-borne disease

Table 5.9 Tasks related to sanitation (disposal of excreta in a rural community)

Collect information	Ascertain the various situations where people dispose of the excreta of adults and of children
	Find out the customs and beliefs related to excreta disposal
	Estimate the extent and seriousness of faecal-borne diseases within the community
Interpret information	Define the main health hazards which result from inadequate faeces disposal
Suggest solutions	From technical knowledge of the types of excreta disposal system, select the type most suitable for the particular community
Start and maintain activities	Explain to the people the health hazards associated with faeces
	Build, with community assistance, a model latrine
	Give technical assistance to families wishing to build latrines
Evaluate	Assess the response of the community in terms of numbers and use of latrines
	Estimate changes in disease patterns over a period of time

Table 5.10 Tasks related to health education within the community

Collect information	Collect information on the knowledge, attitudes and beliefs of the community in relation to particular health patterns Assess the main health problems in terms of frequency, mortality and community concern Identify leaders and opinion formers
Interpret information	Discuss the problems with the people and identify areas of major concern Select for action a priority problem which will respond to health education
Suggest solutions	Define the behavioural change which is needed to improve the health situation Outline a plan for discussing these changes with the people Analyse the factors which might encourage and discourage these changes
Start and maintain activities	Lead group discussion concerning the prevention of disease Devise and use various aids and models (e.g. posters, flipcharts, flannelgraphs) Devise and use other techniques (song, drama, stories, ...)
Evaluate	Assess changes in knowledge and attitude by questionnaire and analysis Estimate change in health status after some time

Table 5.11 Tasks related to treatment of a patient

Collect information	Take a clinical history Conduct a clinical examination of the patient Select and perform special investigations when necessary
Interpret information	Make a provisional diagnosis or Make a definitive diagnosis
Suggest solutions	Write down the patient management Prescribe medicines if necessary Refer, with a letter, when necessary
Start and maintain activities	Explain the management to the patient Explain how to prevent the condition in the future, if relevant Give the prescribed treatment
Evaluate	Check whether the full course of treatment is complete Re-examine the patient to assess improvement

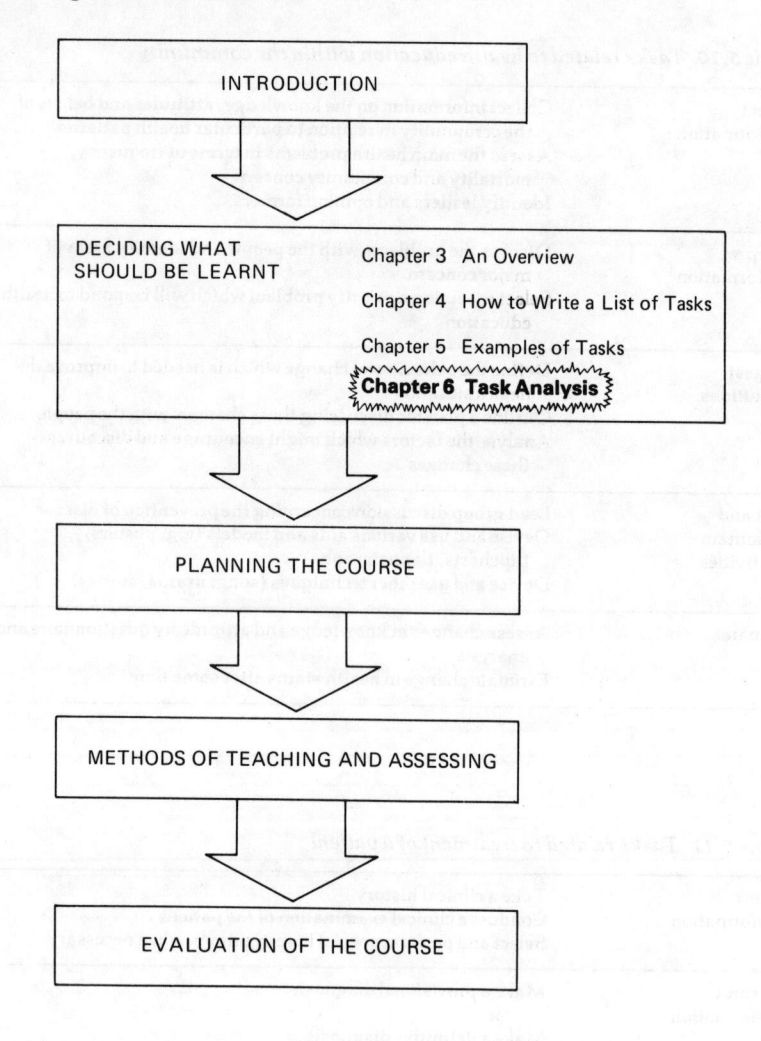

```
        ┌──────────────────┐
        │   INTRODUCTION   │
        └────────┬─────────┘
                 ▼
┌─────────────────────┬──────────────────────────────────┐
│ DECIDING WHAT       │ Chapter 3  An Overview           │
│ SHOULD BE LEARNT    │ Chapter 4  How to Write a List of Tasks │
│                     │ Chapter 5  Examples of Tasks     │
│                     │ Chapter 6  Task Analysis         │
└──────────┬──────────┴──────────────────────────────────┘
           ▼
  ┌────────────────────┐
  │ PLANNING THE COURSE│
  └──────────┬─────────┘
             ▼
  ┌─────────────────────────────────┐
  │ METHODS OF TEACHING AND ASSESSING│
  └──────────────┬──────────────────┘
                 ▼
  ┌─────────────────────────┐
  │ EVALUATION OF THE COURSE│
  └─────────────────────────┘
```

CONTENTS

6.1	Why is Task Analysis Useful?	61
6.2	What do we Mean by a Task Analysis?	63
6.3	How to do a Task Analysis	64
6.4	Defining Relevant and Necessary Knowledge	69
6.5	Conclusion	71

6
Task Analysis

A teacher who has followed the steps outlined in chapter 4, will now have a Task List for his students. This list tells us what students should be able to do at the end of their course. But it does not tell in detail what the teacher should teach to enable the students to do these tasks.

For example, a task might be 'repair a pump for a village well'. What needs to be learnt in order to do this? The process of analysing a task to find out what needs to be learnt is called *task analysis*. The reason for doing a task analysis is

To find out what needs to be learnt in order to do a task

This chapter describes how to analyse tasks.

6.1 WHY IS TASK ANALYSIS USEFUL?

After a teacher has worked very hard at making a task list it would seem to take a lot of work and a great deal of time to do a task analysis on this long list. So we ask the question, is task analysis important? Is it worth while?

Clearly the authors think it is important because we have based five chapters of this book (chapters 10–14) on teaching and assessing the enabling factors and skills derived from task analysis. So before we explain what we mean by task analysis and how to do it, we explain why we think it is important and worthwhile—that is, useful for teaching and learning.

It is not necessary to do a task analysis on every task. This indeed would be laborious and time-consuming. What is needed is a 'task-analysis-way-of-thinking'. Once a teacher develops this way of thinking, he will automatically look for the skills needed when he is training students to do a task.

Task analysis is useful because it clarifies *exactly* what needs to be learnt. From this several advantages may follow:
(1) It makes training more specific. The objectives can be stated in terms of the specific skills a student learns to perform in relation to a task.
(2) The teaching methods needed to help students to learn facts are very different from those needed to help them learn communication or manual skills. By analysing tasks a teacher is able to select teaching methods appropriate to learning the different parts of a task. For example, in learning to palpate a pregnant abdomen it is necessary to give lessons in the classroom on the anatomy of the uterus, to use visual aids (pictures and models) to explain the different positions of

the foetus, and then to practise manual skills on women in the antenatal clinic over a period of time. Different methods are used for teaching the knowledge and the manual skill.

(3) Skills are learned at different speeds. By analysing a task the teacher can plan the allocation of time needed to complete the learning of a task. For example, a community health worker could learn the constituents of a weaning food in about ten minutes (knowledge). But to learn how to prepare it (a manual skill) would take longer and to learn how to explain to mothers its value and how and when to use it (a communication skill) would take longer still.

(4) A task analysis helps us to recognise 'hidden skills'. In the past certain skills have been assumed to be automatically present. It has not been considered possible or necessary to teach them specifically. For example, health workers make decisions all day long—decisions about diagnosis, decisions about treatment, decisions about when to refer a patient, decisions about what to do when supplies run out, when transport breaks down, and so on. Similarly health workers need to communicate—with patients, with their colleagues, with leaders and with villagers. Such skills of decision making and communication have often not been taught specifically in the past. It is now recognised that these two skills—decision making and communication—are of overwhelming importance, particularly in Primary Health Care (PHC). In fact, a PHC worker makes many

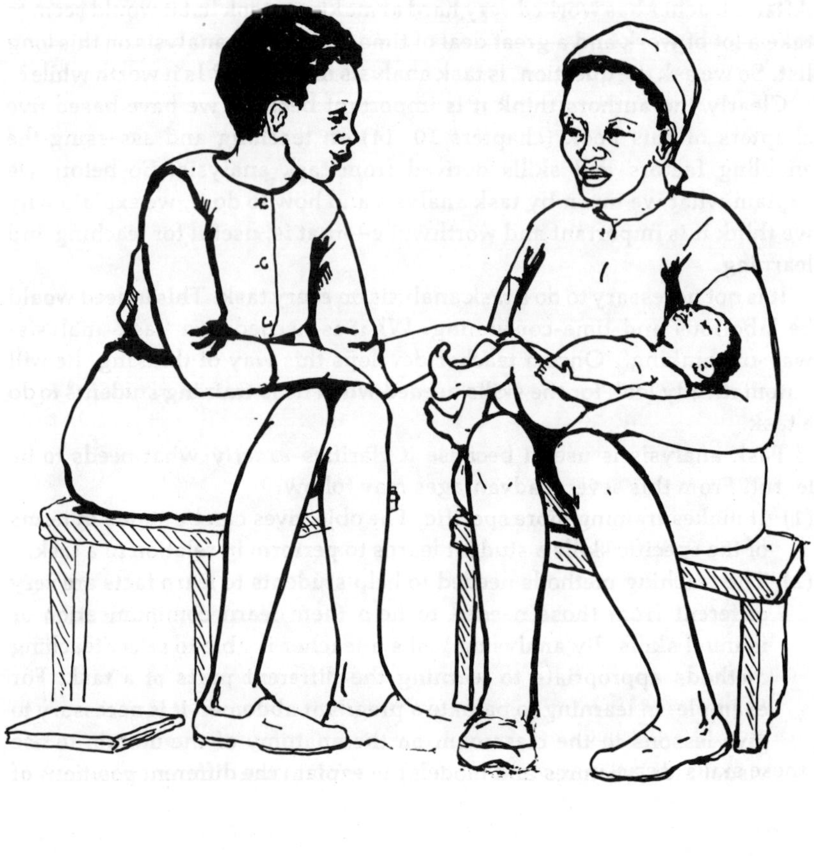

Figure 6.1 The supreme skill needed in Primary Health Care is the ability to communicate well

more decisions than a nurse in a hospital. Nurses normally obey decisions made by the sister or the doctor. Communication is probably more vital to PHC than any other skill. Whereas in hospital-based care the role of the patient is passive, in PHC the health activity is performed by the community. The health worker acts as an information source, as a persuader, as an agent of change within the community.

(5) Doing a task analysis gives a practical rather than theoretical orientation to training. It helps a teacher to think about the actual performance of a task rather than only the knowledge needed to perform it. For example, a health worker may know all the signs and symptoms of leprosy but until he has seen a patient with leprosy he may not recognise them. Task analysis helps a teacher to realise that the task of 'recognising' is not the same as that of 'knowing'.

(6) A task analysis may also be useful as a basis for making a 'checklist', used in the learning and assessment of manual and communication skills. This is described in chapters 12 and 13.

6.2 WHAT DO WE MEAN BY TASK ANALYSIS?

As explained above, task analysis helps a teacher to find out what specific skills are needed by the student to perform a task. Tasks in PHC are of many kinds and come in 'different shapes and sizes'. There are short simple tasks like taking a patient's temperature, complex tasks like examining a patient's chest and long-term tasks like helping a village develop sanitary practices.

Whatever the kind, the complexity or the size of a task, it is usually the case that more than one skill is needed to perform the whole task.

To analyse a task means to:

- examine it carefully in context;
- sub-divide it into its various components (sub-tasks);
- decide which skills are needed to perform it.

How to do this is explained in the next section of this chapter.

Commonly the performance of a task is said to need knowledge, attitude and skills. In this book, rather than just talk about skill, we refer to three different types of skill—these are:

Communication skill
Manual skill
Decision-making skill

Because knowledge and attitude form a necessary background to the performance of any task, we have called these categories 'enabling factors'. They 'enable' the health worker to think about doing the task correctly.

But the actual performance of a task requires more than knowledge and attitude; it will need one or more of the other three skills. We have called these skills 'performance skills'. This is shown diagrammatically below.

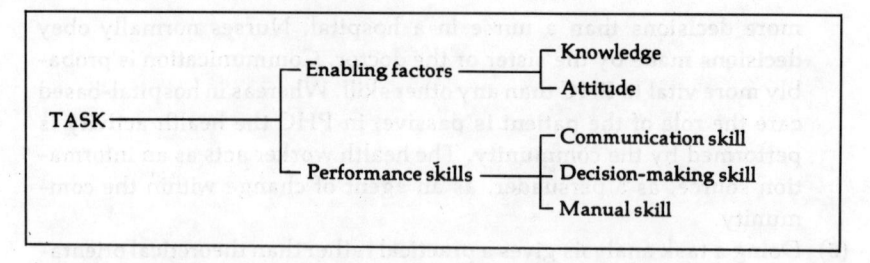

```
                    ┌─ Enabling factors ──┬─ Knowledge
                    │                     └─ Attitude
TASK ───────────────┤
                    │                     ┌─ Communication skill
                    └─ Performance skills ┼─ Decision-making skill
                                          └─ Manual skill
```

Some examples of tasks analysed in this way are shown below.

Two examples of tasks analysed to determine enabling factors and performance skills

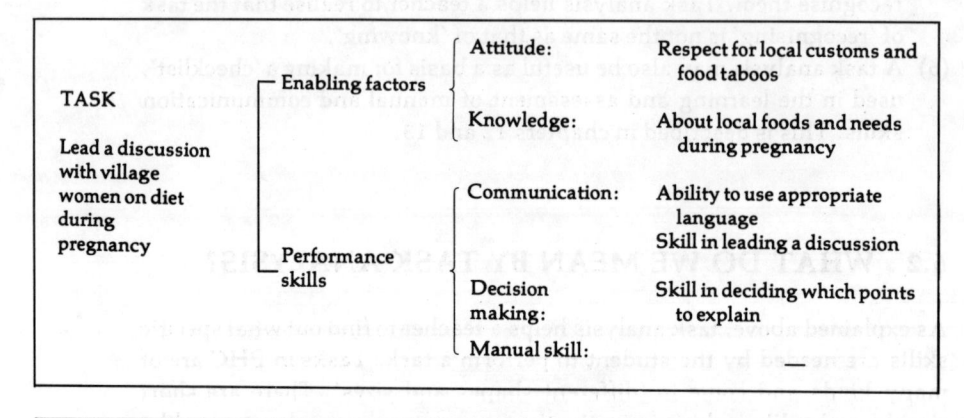

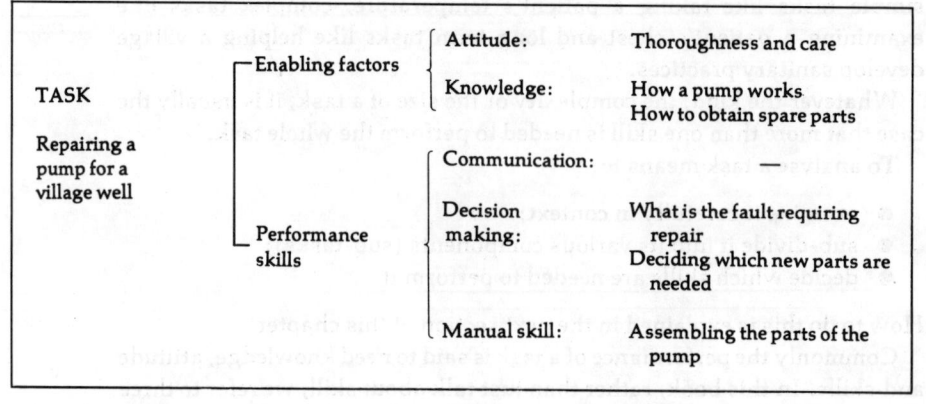

TASK: Lead a discussion with village women on diet during pregnancy

- Enabling factors
  - Attitude: Respect for local customs and food taboos
  - Knowledge: About local foods and needs during pregnancy
- Performance skills
  - Communication: Ability to use appropriate language; Skill in leading a discussion
  - Decision making: Skill in deciding which points to explain
  - Manual skill: —

TASK: Repairing a pump for a village well

- Enabling factors
  - Attitude: Thoroughness and care
  - Knowledge: How a pump works; How to obtain spare parts
- Performance skills
  - Communication: —
  - Decision making: What is the fault requiring repair; Deciding which new parts are needed
  - Manual skill: Assembling the parts of the pump

6.3 HOW TO DO A TASK ANALYSIS

There are three aspects to a complete task analysis:

(i) examine the context;
(ii) divide the tasks into sub-tasks or components;
(iii) define the enabling factors and skills needed.

(i) Examine the Context

This is not always necessary. It is sometimes obvious, but in certain circumstances it is vitally important. By examining the context we mean looking at the situation in which a task will be performed and which facilities/equipment are available.

For example, one task of a health worker may be to sterilise a syringe or a delivery kit. It is well known that there are several ways of sterilising equipment. A hospital will use a steam autoclave, a health centre might use a pressure cooker or an electric dish, a village maternity aid might use a saucepan over a charcoal fire. It is important that health workers learn to do tasks in the context in which they will work using similar equipment and facilities. This is one reason why hospital-based training is inadequate and inappropriate by itself for training primary health care workers.

(ii) Divide the Task into Sub-tasks or Components

To do this a teacher should write down a description of how a person does the task from

- his own memory and experience;
- observing a skilled person performing the task;
- reading up in a book or manual how to do the task;
- discussing with others the components of the task.

From these sources the teacher lists each separate action performed by the person doing the task.

Example

Let us consider a common task performed by most health workers—giving medicine to a patient. Here it is seen how important the context is. Is the task being performed in an outpatients department or in a ward? Are the medicines in liquid form or tablets? Is the patient an adult or a child, literate or illiterate?

Let us look at the sub-tasks of 'giving medicine to a patient' after defining the task context more exactly (table 6.1).

Table 6.1 *Giving one dose of liquid medicine to a young child in a hospital ward*

Sub-tasks or components

Explains to the mother (or guardian) that it is time for the child to receive the medicine
Smiles and talks to the child encouragingly
Asks the mother to place the child on her lap, holding both arms of the child with her left arm
Checks the prescription on the child's chart
Checks the label on the bottle of medicine
Asks the mother to gently open the child's mouth with her right hand by pressing her fingers against the cheeks on each side, while holding the head backwards
Measures out the liquid medicine into a spoon
Quickly tips the liquid through the open mouth
Asks the mother to allow the child to close his mouth
Records on the chart that the medicine has been given

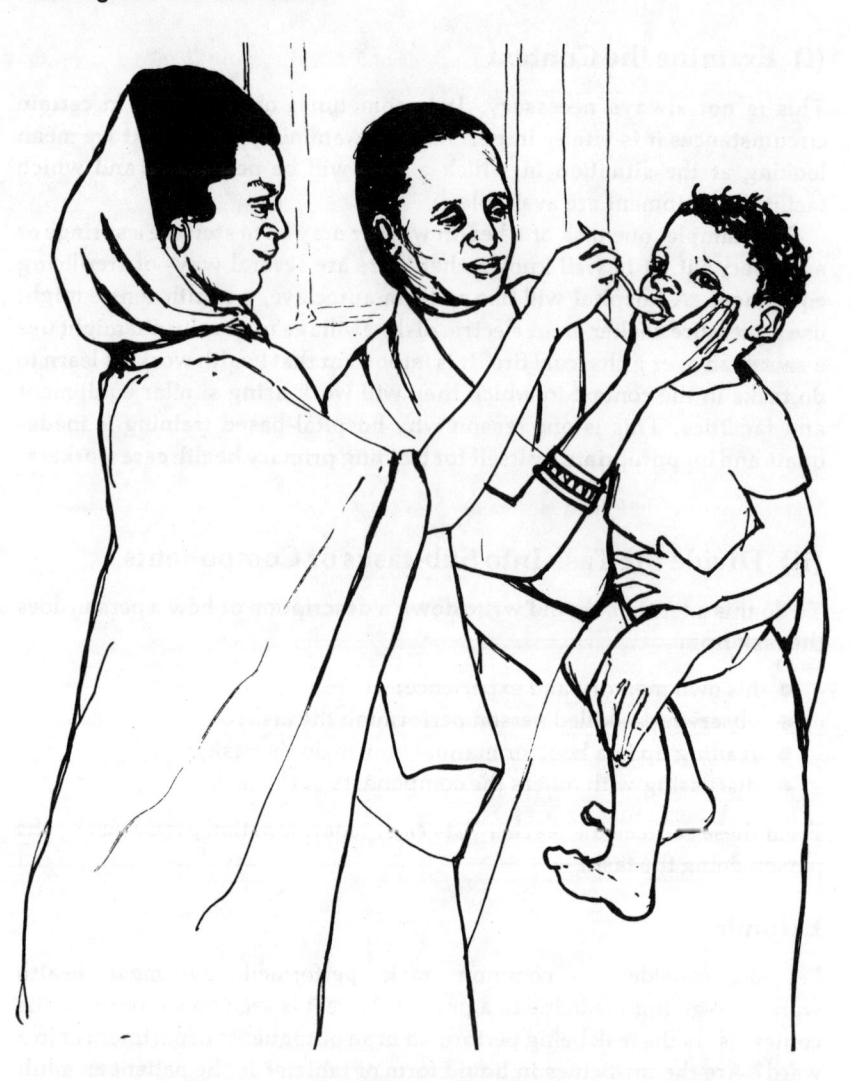

Figure 6.2 Giving liquid medicine to a child in a hospital ward

This example demonstrates that knowledge is not enough. To perform a task well, other skills are needed. Simply to know the correct dose of a medicine is insufficient for the actual performance of the task. Therefore after listing the sub-tasks or components, we need to define the enabling factors and the skills needed.

(iii) Define the Enabling Factors and the Skills

Once the sub-tasks are listed it is a fairly simple process to see which type of skill is required to perform each sub-task. Go through the list and beside each task write the type of skill which seems necessary to perform it.

Alternatively this can be done by means of a table in which the sub-task is written down the left hand vertical column and the type of skills involved are tabulated horizontally. In table 6.2 we do this for the previous example.

Table 6.2 Task: Giving one dose of liquid medicine to a young child in a hospital ward

Sub-tasks	Enabling factors		Performance skills		
	Knowledge	Attitude	Communication	Manual	Decision making
Explains to the mother		✓	✓		
Smiles and talks to the child		✓	✓		
Asks the mother to position the child			✓		
Checks the prescription	✓				
Checks the label	✓				
Asks the mother to open the child's mouth			✓		
Measures out the medicine				✓	
Gives the medicine				✓	
Asks the mother to close the child's mouth			✓		
Records on the chart	✓				

Summary of the Skills Needed to Perform this Task

Knowledge of the best position to hold the child, the names and doses of the medicine and what to record on the chart.

Attitude of friendliness to encourage the child.

Communication with the mother to clearly explain the whole procedure of holding the child and opening his mouth.

Manual skill (very simple) in measuring and delivering the medicine.

Analysis of the Task

'Giving tablets to an illiterate mother at a clinic'

Sub-tasks
Shows the mother one tablet so that she can see its shape and colour
Explains to the mother how this medicine will help her
Asks the mother whether she agrees to take this medicine
Counts out the tablets and puts them in a paper or an envelope
Asks the mother if she has taken tablets before
Explains to the mother how many tablets to take and when
Explains that the medicine will not work in one day but only after the whole course is completed
Puts marks on the paper to remind the mother of the times
Asks the mother to repeat how many tablets to take and when to take them
Tells the mother to return again, if she needs to

What skills does the health worker need to perform this task?

- an *attitude* of respect towards the illiterate mother;
- an *attitude* of patience and willingness to spend time explaining;
- ability to *communicate* effectively with an illiterate person;
- *knowledge* of the tablets, the correct dose and what they are used for;
- a very minor *manual* skill in counting out the tablets

This process may seem to be tedious and to need a great deal of work. Fortunately, it is not necessary to do this in detail for every single task. Once a teacher grasps the general idea behind the procedure he will rapidly pick out the components and skills involved in any given task. In the example given above, the skills are shown directly below the list of sub-tasks, the stage of tabulation has been omitted. (Giving tablets to an illiterate mother at a clinic.)

There is another reason why it is not necessary to do a task analysis for every task. There are certain types of tasks which have a repetitive pattern. An analysis of one task within a group will reveal the skills required for the whole group. Clinical skills are an example of this. In the broad area of clinical diagnosis, patient management and patient education we find three performance skills constantly recurring. These skills are summarised below.

(1) Communicating

Interviewing the patient to elicit the history.
Reassuring the patient during examination.
Explaining to the patient why investigations are necessary.
Explaining the proposed management to the patient.
Finding out what the patient already knows.
Explaining to the patient how to prevent a future recurrence.

(2) Decision making

Deciding what questions to ask.
Deciding which part of the history is significant.
Deciding whether a sign is normal or abnormal.
Deciding the diagnosis or provisional diagnosis.
Deciding on the management.
Deciding the appropriate dose of drug.
Deciding which investigations are needed.

(3) Manual Skills

Conducting the whole range of clinical and physical examinations.
Conducting investigations.
Doing clinical procedures.
Doing major or minor operative procedures.

A teacher who thinks in a task analysis way will constantly ask himself these questions:

- What manual skills are necessary to do this?
- At what point are decisions made during this task?
- Will this task be done better if the health worker can communicate well?

But, although defining performance skills from a task component list is usually straightforward, the amount of 'knowledge' needed for a particular task needs further thought.

6.4 DEFINING RELEVANT AND NECESSARY KNOWLEDGE

The success of the health worker in his performance of tasks will depend on his knowledge being relevant to the job. But even if we say 'select the knowledge needed to perform the task' the answer is not easy. Which knowledge is really necessary and how much?

When a task is described accurately and a task analysis has been done the knowledge relevant to the task should become clear. This will help a teacher to define the minimal and necessary knowledge but it will not of itself answer the question 'how much'?

There are two main reasons why the question 'how much' presents so much difficulty (and also disagreement among educators).

(i) One reason for this difficulty is that knowledge has functions related to the performance of a wider range of tasks—such as deciding priorities and making judgements.

As a general principle we can say

> A health worker needs the knowledge necessary to make rational decisions and judgements about his work

In applying this principle the amount of knowledge needed will depend on the level of responsibility attached to the task. The description of a task needs to be accurate enough to indicate the level of responsibility required.

The example in table 6.3 illustrates this principle. Each health worker has tasks related to anaemia in pregnancy but the tasks require different levels of skill and responsibility. Therefore the amount of knowledge required in each case will be different. It should be noted that the knowledge required for 'higher' levels of skill, includes that required for 'simpler' levels. The medical assistant needs the knowledge of both the MCH aide and the community nurse.

It can be seen from this example that the more clearly a task is defined, the easier it becomes to determine the relevant knowledge.

(ii) Another reason why it is difficult to decide how much knowledge is needed, is that knowledge has an important value for the individual in creating interest, satisfying curiosity and understanding the world.

It is sometimes said against the task analysis approach that it deprives the learner of his basic right to wide, deep and broad knowledge! If this were true, it would be a reasonable objection. No person should prevent others from learning. No teacher can be justified in confining students to minimal knowledge.

We agree that each person should know as much as possible about his work. But we think that before he learns 'as much as possible', he should learn 'what is essential to do the job'.

Relevant knowledge defines what *every* student *must know* in order to do his job well. Relevant knowledge defines the Core of

Essential Knowledge. After this core has been achieved teachers and students may expand knowledge as widely as their interests lead them.

This idea has been expressed as the Target Concept. This divides knowledge into three categories—must know, helpful to know and nice to know.

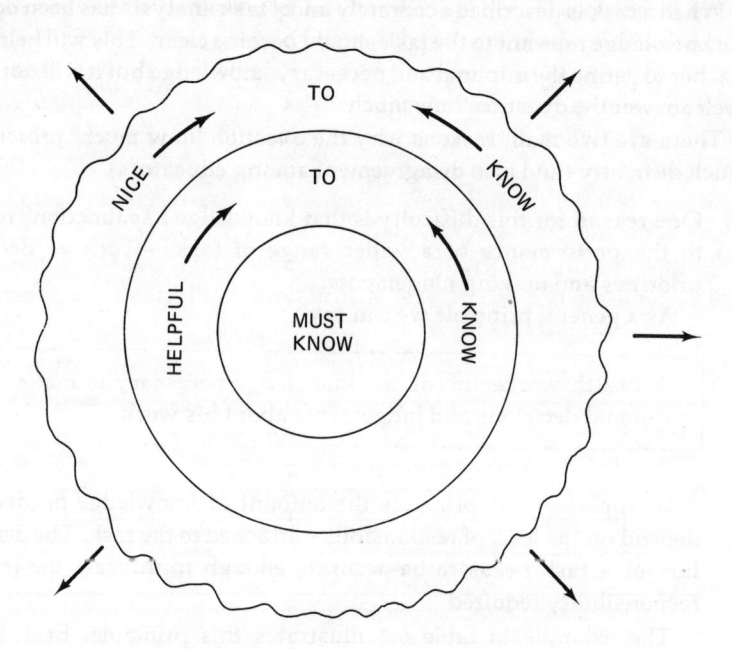

Table 6.3 *How the amount of knowledge needed about 'anaemia in pregnancy' varies with the level of health worker*

Health worker	Task	Knowledge needed
MCH Aide in a village	Treat pregnant women for clinical anaemia	Dangers of anaemia in pregnancy Local foods containing iron Dosage of iron tablets
Community nurse in a Health Centre	Treat pregnant women for clinical anaemia Refer when necessary	*As above,* plus Knowledge of several causes of anaemia Doses of iron and folic acid Treatment of hookworm and malaria Knowledge of levels of anaemia in relation to the stages of pregnancy
Medical Assistant in charge of an area	Recognise the prevalence of anaemia in pregnancy in his area Advise on prevention	*As above,* plus Knowledge of simple survey methods Knowledge of possible factors associated with high prevalence Knowledge of preventive measures available against main factors—such as Hookworm, Malaria, Malnutrition

6.5 CONCLUSION

We have seen that a task Analysis helps teachers to decide what skills need to be taught for health workers to perform their job well. It also helps to decide how much knowledge is necessary for successful health work.

In fact the Task Analysis completes the process of 'Deciding what should be learnt'. The list of knowledge and attitude, together with the list of the three types of skill is a *complete* list of what should be learnt, or— as some teachers would describe it—a complete list of the *objectives* for the course.

What follows from this is that the task analysis also determines what should be included in the assessment of the students. Students should not be assessed on knowledge or skills which do not appear in any of the task analyses. But they should be assessed on as wide a range as possible of the items in the task analyses.

This is a vitally important stage to complete. If it is done well, the course has a good chance of success; if it is done badly then the course will inevitably be unsatisfactory.

SUMMARY

- Task analysis helps to make training more specific and guides the choice of teaching methods.
- Task analysis is done in 3 stages
    (i) examining the context in which the task is performed;
    (ii) listing each stage in performing the task, i.e. the sub-tasks;
    (iii) deciding what types of skill are involved and what knowledge and attitudes are required.
- The outcome of the task analysis is a complete list of what the students should learn—and a complete list of what should be assessed.

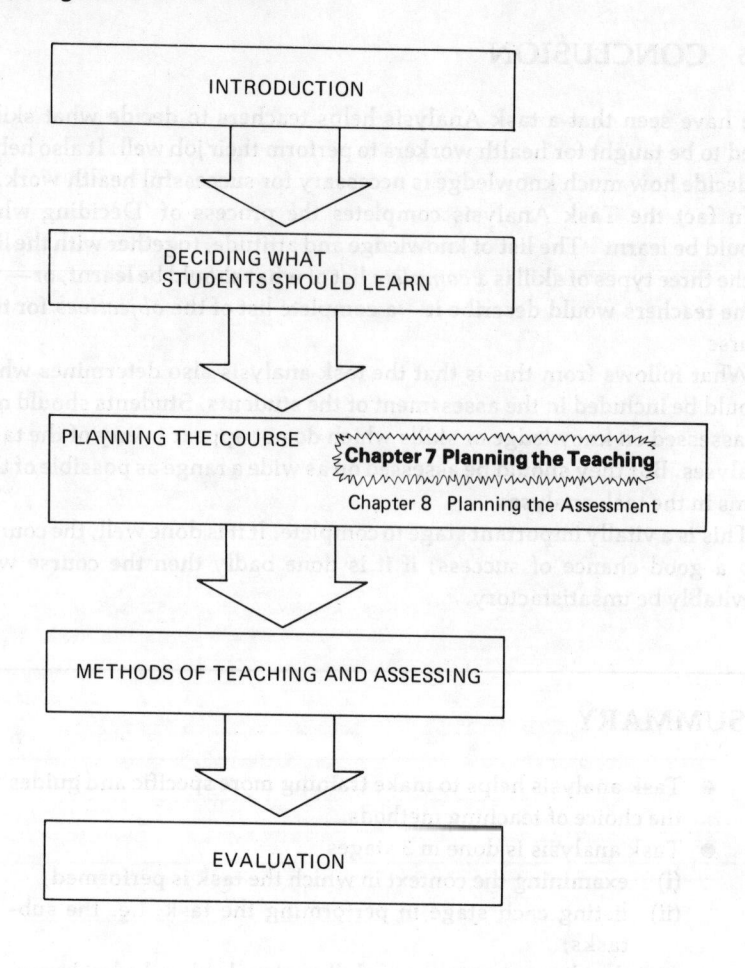

```
           ┌──────────────────┐
           │   INTRODUCTION   │
           └──────────────────┘
                    │
                    ▼
           ┌──────────────────┐
           │   DECIDING WHAT  │
           │ STUDENTS SHOULD LEARN │
           └──────────────────┘
                    │
                    ▼
           ┌──────────────────┐
           │ PLANNING THE COURSE │   **Chapter 7 Planning the Teaching**
           │                  │   Chapter 8  Planning the Assessment
           └──────────────────┘
                    │
                    ▼
           ┌──────────────────────────────┐
           │ METHODS OF TEACHING AND ASSESSING │
           └──────────────────────────────┘
                    │
                    ▼
           ┌──────────────────┐
           │    EVALUATION    │
           └──────────────────┘
```

CONTENTS

7.1	Grouping the Task List	73
7.2	Planning a Course Programme	74
7.3	Why is it Important to Plan a Course Programme?	74
7.4	How to Plan a Course Programme	75
7.5	Example of a Course Programme	76
7.6	Planning a Lesson	78
7.7	Planning Practical Work and Field Visits	82
7.8	Review	83

7
Planning the Teaching

So far, by means of a Task List and Task Analysis we have defined what is to be taught.

We now have to arrange the contents (knowledge and skills) into a course programme. This means that the knowledge and skills to be learnt must be fitted into the time allowed for the course and arranged in the places and according to the facilities available for teaching.

This organisation of course content involves:

(1) Grouping the Task List (section 7.1).
(2) Planning a course programme (sections 7.2–7.5).
(3) Planning practical work and field visits (section 7.7).
(4) Planning a lesson (section 7.6).

This scheme only deals with planning the teaching for a single course, that is a short complete course or a course within a larger multi-course training programme. Planning a complete training programme which involves several courses is beyond the scope of this book.

7.1 GROUPING THE TASK LIST

Before arranging a course programme or planning the individual lessons it is necessary to group the tasks under convenient headings. There is no one single correct way to group tasks. But it is more convenient to teach and learn tasks which are grouped into areas of activity which are related. Convenience and relatedness are the main criteria a teacher can use in grouping the task list.

For example, there is little difficulty in arranging tasks in maternal care. The tasks group themselves naturally:

- caring for mothers in the antenatal period;
- caring for mothers during delivery;
- caring for mothers in the postnatal period;
- advising mothers on health, family planning and nutrition;
- caring for the newborn.

Grouping of tasks in the way suggested relates directly to the job of the Primary Health Care (PHC) worker and makes learning more meaningful and more easily applied.

We do not think the old-fashioned way of learning according to subjects is useful for PHC workers. We believe that learning basic topics like anatomy, pathology and microbiology is more meaningful and more easily applied when it is learned in relation to a task. For example, the anatomy of bones and joints can be learned in relation to the management of fractures and dislocations. Microbiology is learned in relation to sterilisation and infectious conditions. In this way the relevant and necessary knowledge is task-related and is less likely to be forgotten.

If the course is a long one, then there will be a need for smaller groups of tasks under the main groupings. For example, antenatal care could be sub-divided into tasks related to diagnosis in early pregnancy, bleeding during pregnancy, detecting the at-risk patients and so on. A further example of sub-dividing task groups is shown under section 7.2 Planning a Course Programme. This example sub-divides the tasks of immunising young children.

There are several ways in which clinical tasks can be grouped. Some teachers group tasks according to the presenting symptom, for example, cough, diarrhoea, fever, headache and so on. Another convenient grouping for clinical tasks is according to body systems—that is conditions relating to the respiratory system, the digestive system and so on.

Although there is no one single correct way to group tasks, it must be remembered that learning will be enhanced if the grouping makes sense to the student and follows a logical sequence. The way information is presented to a student is likely to be way in which he remembers it and associates it for the rest of his life. For this reason, whatever grouping is chosen it should be logical and coherent.

7.2 PLANNING A COURSE PROGRAMME

By the word 'course' we are referring to a distinct topic (a group of tasks) arranged by one teacher over a definite length of time, such as a term or a year. The 'topic' might be a subject such as microbiology but it would be better if it was a group of tasks, such as caring for mothers or looking after sick children or establishing a water supply. What each individual course contains will depend on the grouping of the task list and on the task analysis.

By the word 'Programme' we mean when and where different tasks will be taught. Teaching tasks takes place during class periods, practical sessions, field visits, self-study periods and assessment periods. The course programme arranges the learning experiences in time and place.

7.3 WHY IS IT IMPORTANT TO PLAN A COURSE PROGRAMME?

There are several reasons why planning ahead improves both teaching and learning.

(a) It is the only way in which time given to various sections of the course can be balanced. Failure to plan usually results in 'cramming' at the end because insufficient time is left to finish learning all the tasks.
(b) Structure is an important factor in learning. It is easier to learn a topic

which is well arranged so that one topic follows another in a logical sequence (see chapter 9).

(c) A teacher cannot plan and prepare lessons ahead of time unless he has a course programme.

(d) As far as possible, performance skills of a task need to be practised as soon as the enabling factors have been absorbed. A course programme helps a teacher to arrange practicals which relate to knowledge learnt.

(e) Field visits need to be arranged well in advance and should fit into the teaching programme.

(f) If continuous assessment needs to be part of the course, this also needs to be planned in advance—so that there is good sampling of the course when assessing the students' skills (see chapter 8).

(g) If the course programme is given to the students they will experience a sense of progress as they learn.

7.4 HOW TO PLAN A COURSE PROGRAMME

(i) There are so many columns needed for a course programme plan that is is necessary to join two sheets of paper together with sellotape (or alternatively use double foolscap if it is available). You will need 7 columns and the columns 4, 5, and 7 should be wide.

The column headings are shown in the diagram.

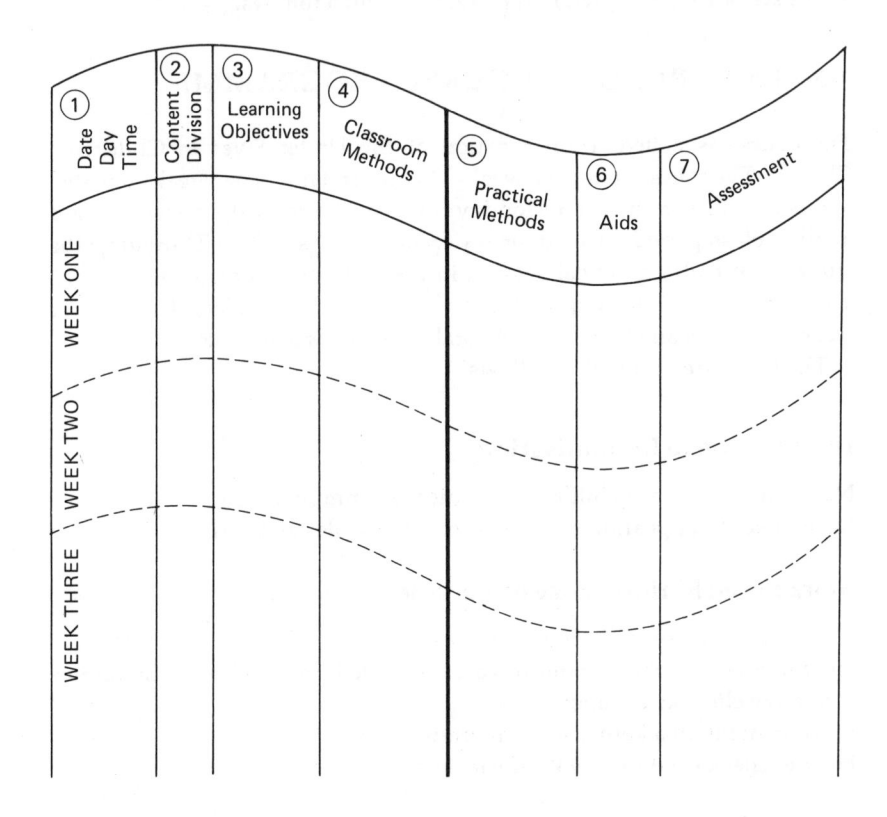

① Date Day Time	② Content Division	③ Learning Objectives	④ Classroom Methods	⑤ Practical Methods	⑥ Aids	⑦ Assessment
WEEK ONE						
WEEK TWO						
WEEK THREE						

(ii) Now study the time you have available to teach the tasks. If you are working with a timetable prepared by a Principal or Head Teacher you will have been allocated a certain number of class periods and some practical sessions (clinic, ward or laboratory) during a period of a number of weeks the course will last.

If you are making your own timetable, you will need to decide how much time to give to classes and practicals.

(iii) In the left hand column of your programme sheets, write the date, day, time of all the classes week by week, down the column.

(iv) Next divide the tasks in your course into groups and spread the groups down column 2, allocating a definite number of sessions to each group of tasks.

(v) In column 3 write the objectives of each lesson, i.e. the knowledge, skills and attitudes which will be learnt.

(vi) Columns 4 and 5 summarise the main teaching method you will use. That is the learning experience which will help to achieve the objectives. These chosen methods will later be elaborated into full lesson plans (see Planning a Lesson).

(vii) If any teaching aids will be needed, write these in column 6. This is particularly important if aids need to be borrowed or prepared beforehand.

(viii) In column 7 write down the assessments which you plan. These may refer to class tests, record or log books, checklists or final examinations.

These steps are illustrated in the example which follows.

7.5 EXAMPLE OF A COURSE PROGRAMME

The course is called 'Immunisation of the Under Fives in Childrens' Clinics'. The course lasts for 6 weeks. There are 4 hours per week allocated to this course. One hour on Monday from 8 to 9 a.m. in the classroom and another class period on Wednesday from 9 to 10 a.m. On Thursdays the students attend a practical session in the childrens' clinic from 10 to 12 a.m. The teacher designing this programme has therefore 4 hours per week, 2 in class and 2 in clinic. A total of 24 hours in 6 weeks.

The tasks are grouped as follows.

Introduction to Immunisation

Name the diseases of children prevented by immunisation.
Recognise the appearance of the vaccine ampoules and vials.

Storage and Maintenance of Vaccines

How to fill in an order form for vaccines.
How to calculate the amount of vaccine needed from the child population and the clinic attendance.
How to maintain a kerosene refrigerator.
How to check existing stocks of vaccines.

Giving Immunisation

The dosage schedule of immunisation and how to administer the vaccines.
The contraindications—recognising when not to give vaccine.

Educating Mothers and the Community

How to communicate with mothers the importance of immunisation.
Explaining the side effects to mothers.

From this grouping, the programme can be arranged within the six week period as shown in table 7.1.

7.6 PLANNING A LESSON

After a teacher has made an outline of his programme he can then start to plan each lesson in detail.

The lesson is the focus where the teacher's skill is applied.

The teacher's understanding of what helps people learn and his skill in using techniques suited to particular types of learning is given practical expression in the lesson.

The educational circle (shown in the diagram), applies to every lesson, as well as to the teaching programme as a whole.

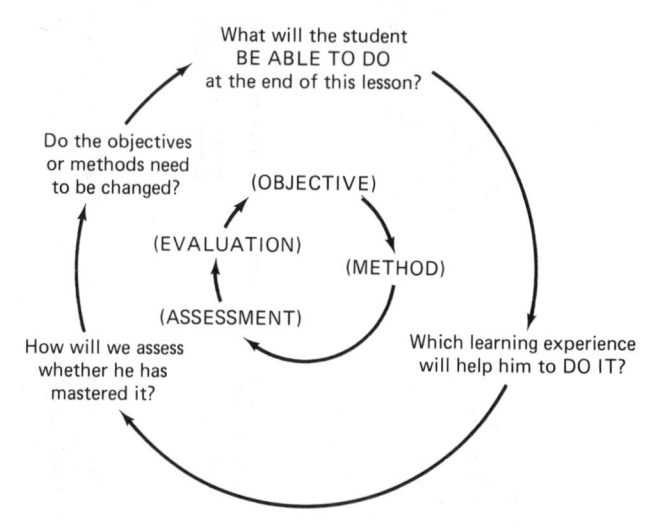

Diagram: Educational circle showing inner cycle of (OBJECTIVE) → (METHOD) → (ASSESSMENT) → (EVALUATION) → back to (OBJECTIVE); and outer cycle with questions: "What will the student BE ABLE TO DO at the end of this lesson?", "Which learning experience will help him to DO IT?", "How will we assess whether he has mastered it?", "Do the objectives or methods need to be changed?"

In *planning* a lesson we can go through a systematic scheme which helps us to answer these questions. There are several schemes which can be used—but whatever scheme is used the above questions should be clearly answered.

By *preparation* of a lesson we mean collecting and making the resources needed by the plan which has been outlined. For example, handouts, models, visual aids, tests and exercises.

Planning and preparing lessons takes a great amount of a teacher's time. There are some compensations.

Table 7.1

Date	Day	Time	Division of topic	Learning objectives	Classroom methods	Practical methods	Aids	Assessment
Week One	Mon	8–9	Introduction to immunisation	Name diseases which immunisation can prevent	Lesson and handout		Handout	
	Wed	9–10		Recognise the vaccine ampoules	Demonstration in the class. Class handles the vaccines		Example of each type used	
	Thurs	10–11 11–12		Observe and describe clinic routine		Observation in the clinic followed by questions and discussion		
Week Two	Mon	8–9	Storage and maintenance of vaccines	How to complete an order form Calculation of amount necessary	Exercises with examples		Order forms	
	Wed	9–10			Different exercises using different populations			
	Thurs	10–11				Examination of working refrigerator		Record book to record observations
		11–12				Assist in clinic work		
Week Three	Mon	8–9		How to maintain a kerosene fridge	Diagram of model in class		Diagram handout	
	Wed	9–10		Checking procedure when not in good working order	Lesson on faults and repairs			
	Thurs	10–11 11–12		How to store vaccines in the fridge		Observe methods of storage Assist with giving vaccines		Record book to record vaccines given

Planning the Teaching

	Time	Area	Topic	Method / Activity	Assessment / Materials
Week Four					
Mon	8–9	Giving immunisation	TEST		Class test on learning of first 2 weeks
	9–10		National immunisation schedule		
	10–11			Continue practising giving immunisations in the clinic	Record book
	11–12				
Wed			When *not* to give	Handout to learn lesson (brief); Lesson on contraindications	Handout
Thurs					
Week Five					
Mon	8–9	Educating mothers and community	How to communicate with mothers	Discussion of mothers' attitude found by previous clinic experience	
Wed	9–10				
Thurs	11–12			Practise talking with mothers in very small groups	
Week Six					
Mon	8–9		Explaining side effects to mothers	Discussion on side effects seen so far in the clinic. Discussion on best approach. Role play	
Wed	9–10		How to conduct a home visit		
Thurs	10–11	Assessment period			Written test (brief) Practical exercises Checklist assessment on technique of injection
	11–12				

- The students learn better and the class atmosphere improves.
- Plans and resources used this year can be used again—so useful material is gradually built up.
- Planning lessons becomes a habit of thought and gets quicker with practice.

Outline of a Lesson-planning Process

(i) Review the context of the lesson
   Time, space, resources, students, place in the course programme
(ii) Define the objective
(iii) Plan the introduction
(iv) Plan the learning strategies
   (a) Analyse the skills component of the objective.
   (b) Select a teaching strategy suitable for the skill.
   (c) Think of resources needed to support the strategy.
   (d) Divide the activities into within the lesson and outside the lesson period.
   (e) Write out the lesson procedure sequence.
(v) Plan the summary.
(vi) Plan the follow-up.
(vii) Plan the assessment.

(i) Review the Context of the Lesson

Do not take a particular teaching situation for granted. See if it can be improved.

Time	The commonest mistake in teaching is cramming too much learning into too short a time. Can the time be increased? If not, reduce the objectives of the course or the lesson.
Space	Be imaginative. Don't assume the classroom is the only place to teach. There may be an empty shed, an unused laboratory, a local building, a verandah or a tree—where you can spread out your class for group work or practicals.
Resources	Make efforts to increase your teaching aids—use local materials, make your own models, posters, photographs, use student artists to draw your visual aids, contact local charities or agencies to buy/give you equipment.
Students	Review the level and number of your students. Numbers of students affect the types of methods which are feasible.
Course programme	Every lesson needs to be connected into a coherent programme. Review what has preceded this lesson and what will follow.

(ii) Define the Objectives

Every planned lesson must have an objective or objectives. If not it is an unplanned lesson.

The difficulty in defining the objective is related to time. The objective must be something which can be learned within the period allocated for the lesson. If the particular task being learned covers a period of several lessons then the task needs to be broken up into components.

For example,   Task: To be able to treat a dehydrated child
Lesson 1   Objective: To recognise the symptoms and signs of dehydration and decide whether it is moderate or severe.
Lesson 2   Objective: To identify dehydrated children requiring intravenous fluid and to refer.
Lesson 3   Objective: To be able to make oral rehydration mixture
— in a clinic
— in a home
and give to the child in correct quantities.

> Define the objectives for every lesson

Know where you and the students are going!

(iii) Plan the Introduction

Refer to previous experience or to a previous lesson in the course. Remind the students by open questions about their experience or what they remember from previous lessons.

Introduce the objective in some way. Explain the direction and goal and meaning of the lesson.

Emphasise *relevance*. This may be done by:

- telling a story;
- explaining problems which the lesson may solve;
- giving examples of application of the new learning;
- asking questions which bring out the relevance.

Indicate how and when the lesson will be assessed.

(iv) Plan the Learning Strategies

A teaching technique or a learning experience needs to be suited to the skill to be learned. This is obvious in some cases. For example, you cannot learn to ride a bicycle by listening to a lecture or attending a film. Similarly, you cannot learn to deliver a baby in a classroom.

(a) *Analyse the Skills Component in the Lesson Objective*

How to analyse tasks and derive the necessary component skills has been explained in detail in chapter 6.

After defining the objective to be achieved within the lesson, a teacher should decide which type of skill or skills the student needs to learn to achieve the objective.

The teaching method/learning experience will be chosen according to the skills needed.

(b) Select a Teaching Strategy Suitable for the Skill

In chapters 10–14 approaches to teaching different types of skill are discussed in detail.

To help teachers in the selection of methods, a summary of teaching methods related to skills is given at the end of chapter 9 (see table 9.1).

(c) Think of the Resources Needed to Support the Strategy

These may be stories, examples, illustrations, visual aids, models, exercises, handouts and so on.

(d) Divide the Activities

The activities needed to learn the objective may be done within the lesson period. But very often, because of time constraints, some activities are continued or completed outside the lesson—as homework, during a practical, during a roster in a clinic or ward. The relation of the future activity to this lesson should be made clear to the student.

(e) Write out the Lesson Procedure in Sequence

This is a help in putting the learning strategies in logical order and also in assessing the time required for each stage of the lesson (see table 7.2).

Table 7.2 A model outline of a lesson plan

Objective		Time	
Students should be able to describe the life-cycle of the malaria parasite		1 h	
Introduction			
1. Refer to previous lesson—causes of fever		2 min	
2. Malaria—a worldwide and national problem		3 min	
3. Understanding cycle helps treatment and control		3 min	
Content	*Teacher activity*		*Student Activity*
The cycle in general	Gives diagrammatic handout with names of main stages	2 min	
		5 min	Students read handout
The stages in detail	Shows slides (or posters) of each stage one at a time Explains details of each stage	5 min per stage	
	Asks students to draw each stage	5 min per stage	Students draw
Summary	Shows slides again and asks students to write down names as they appear	8 min	Students write names
Assessment	Collects the papers	2 min	
Follow-up			
Arranges microscope and mosquito demonstrations in the laboratory			

(v) Plan the Summary

There are many ways in which a teacher can summarise a lesson:
- ask the class to say what they have learned;
- review the main points;
- ask pertinent questions;
- summarise in a handout;
- put up a transparency/or write on the blackboard.

(vi) Plan the Follow-up

Most lessons need to be followed up by the students to consolidate their learning by:
- reading and learning the handout;
- looking up references in a manual or a library;
- doing exercises/project work;
- practising during clinics/field work.

(vii) Plan the Assessment

Assessment during the lesson:
- give exercises to be handed back;
- observe while practical work is taking place;
- assess group work and discussion;
- ask a rapid series of questions.

Assessment later.
At the end of every lesson prepare an assessment to test that particular objective. It might be:
- a multiple-choice question;
- a short-answer question;
- a checklist;
- a project.

Keep these to be used in a weekly test, a continuous assessment programme or an end of course examination.

7.7 PLANNING PRACTICAL WORK AND FIELD VISITS

Practical training for students of primary health care may include:
- community surveys;
- educational visits;
- home-visiting;
- field practicals (e.g. building latrines);
- clinic work;
- ward work;
- laboratory work;
- giving health talks or nutrition demonstrations.

For the teacher, planning the practical work in a course is even more time-consuming than planning and preparing lessons.

After making a list of all the practical experiences which the students need it is convenient to divide the list into two groups:

(1) Events which may occur once only.
(2) Practicals which occur weekly throughout the timetable.

The rotating of students through situations in which they practise manual and other procedures is described in detail in chapter 9. The many difficulties experienced by teachers in making these arrangements have also been discussed.

Here we are concerned with planning single events, such as a survey or an educational visit. Because such visits are often to villages, or to distant places, they usually involve people outside the health field or outside the Government and need to be planned well in advance.

Planning a Field Visit

(a) Make sure that there is a clear learning objective to the visit and that it is worthwhile. Since field visits need a great deal of preparation and often cost money, the learning derived from the experience should be valuable.
(b) Find out the cheapest transport available and book it in advance, if necessary. Usually, sending students on local buses or vans is the cheapest.
(c) Visit the site well in advance and interview the people who will be receiving the students. In the case of a village this might be the village head or council or the village health committee. In the case of a visit to a water development scheme it might be an official of a local government department.
(d) If the students are staying overnight, arrange for their accommodation and food.
(e) Develop a project-form related to the visit. This might be a questionnaire in the case of a survey or it might be a series of questions which the students will answer after making observations during the visit.
(f) Just before the appointed date, contact those who will receive the students to remind them of the visit. Check that the transport, accommodation and food arrangements are in order.
(g) Explain to the students the purpose of the visit and what they will be expected to do.
(h) Review the visit, after returning, to make sure that students have learned from the experience. Consolidate and reinforce the learning.

7.8 REVIEW

At this point, a major part of ensuring that a course will train PHC workers effectively has been achieved.

The content of the course has been selected to include all the important enabling objectives and performance objectives. Also all the trivia and unimportant information should have been excluded from the content, so that students can concentrate on those things which matter. If this has been done well, there is a very good chance that the course will correspond closely to the needs of the health service and the needs of communities which are served.

The overall structure of the course—and of the lessons within the course—will have been planned in a logical way. This will help students to learn and will ensure that there is about the right amount of time available for each part of the course. These two achievements are very substantial and important. If they are not carried out well, there is no prospect of the course being successful.

From this point the book goes on to consider how the course assessment can be planned. Then the teaching methods that are available will be considered in chapters 9–14.

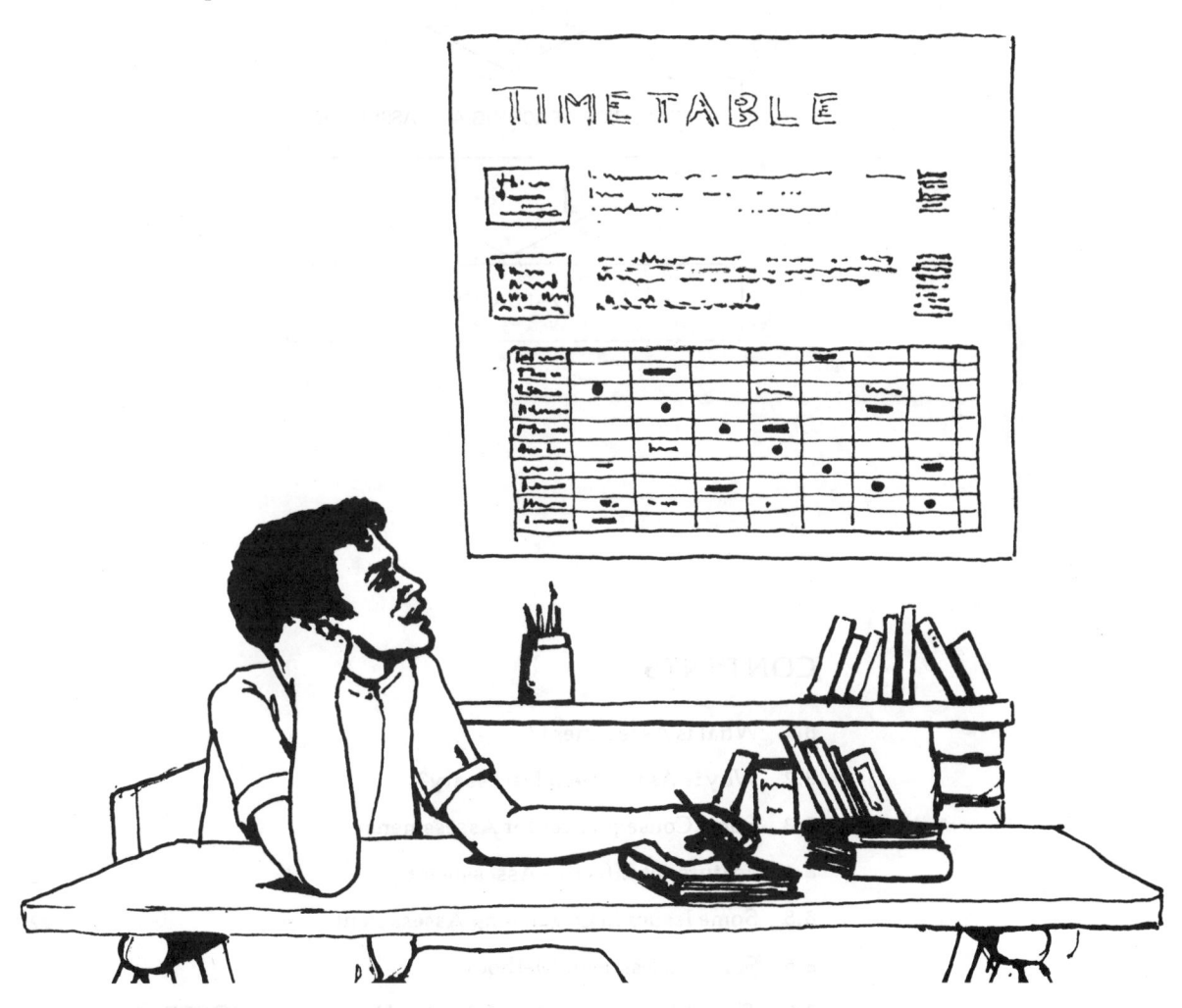

Figure 7.1 Planning a course well is a major achievement: all that is left to be done is to do the teaching!

```
        ┌─────────────────┐
        │  INTRODUCTION   │
        └────────┬────────┘
                 ▼
        ┌─────────────────────────────┐
        │ DECIDING WHAT SHOULD BE LEARNT │
        └────────┬────────────────────┘
                 ▼
        ┌──────────────────────────────────────────────┐
        │ PLANNING THE COURSE   Chapter 7  Planning the Teaching │
        │                       **Chapter 8 Planning the Assessment** │
        └────────┬─────────────────────────────────────┘
                 ▼
        ┌──────────────────────────────┐
        │ METHODS OF TEACHING AND ASSESSING │
        └────────┬─────────────────────┘
                 ▼
        ┌─────────────────┐
        │   EVALUATION    │
        └─────────────────┘
```

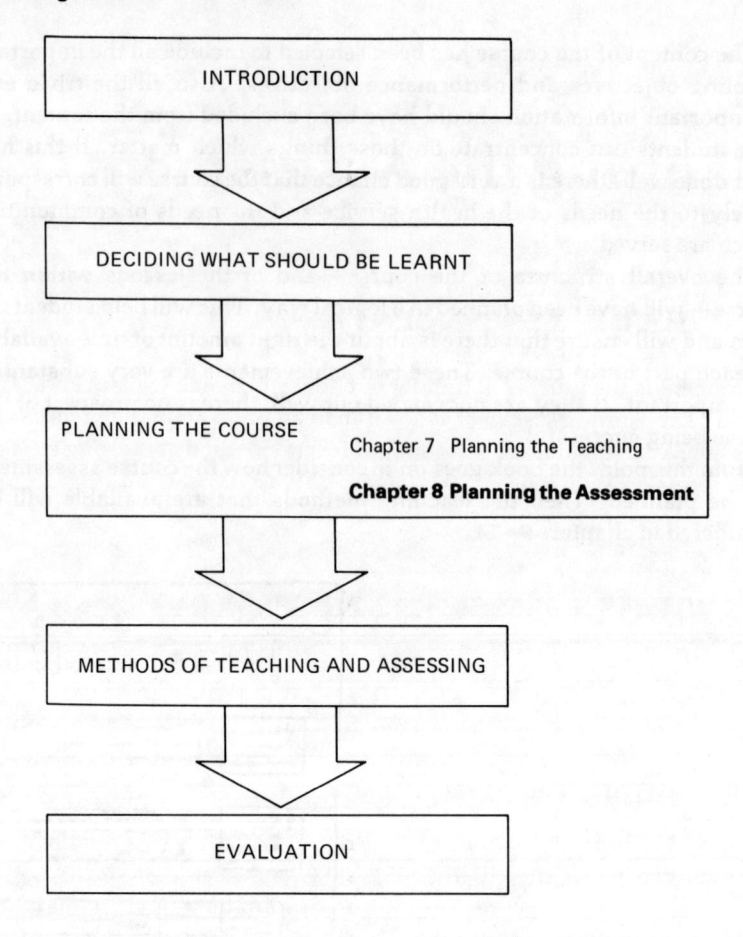

CONTENTS

8.1	What is Assessment?	87
8.2	Why is Assessment Necessary?	87
8.3	Some Consequences for Assessment	88
8.4	Features of Effective Assessment	90
8.5	Some Issues in Organising Assessment	92
8.6	Some Assessment Methods	94
8.7	The Objective Structured Practical Examination (OSPE)	94

8
Planning the Assessment

8.1 WHAT IS ASSESSMENT?

Assessment is the process of finding out how much each student knows or can do. The word assessment is used instead of 'examinations' because assessment can include all sorts of less formal methods of testing as well as the formal examination.

8.2 WHY IS ASSESSMENT NECESSARY?

There are three main reasons why students should be assessed. These are as follows.

(i) To Certify the Student

In all types of health care, the health care workers can save or prolong life and they can make the environment safer and healthier. But if health workers are incompetent, they can kill or injure patients and can make the environment more dangerous. So there is a clear need to make sure that every health worker is sufficiently competent to be of benefit to the community before he or she is allowed to practise as a recognised health worker. This process of certifying a student as competent to provide health care is one of the key functions of assessment.

(ii) To Guide Students and Teachers

During a course students may have failed to understand an idea or failed to reach a suitable standard of skill. Ideally they should realise this weakness as soon as possible so that they can work to remedy their specific weaknesses.

Similarly, a teacher may have confused most of the students in a group or may have taught a skill in such a way that the students are still not competent. Again it would be valuable if the teacher realised that things had gone wrong so that the lesson could be taught again in such a way that the errors could be corrected.

In both these examples, regular assessment can be used to detect what teaching or learning had to be repeated and so provide guidance to both students and teachers. Assessment can in this way provide some 'quality control' and so help to improve the quality of both teaching and learning.

(iii) To Motivate Students and Teachers

Assessment can provide an extra stimulus to both students and teachers and in this way encourage learning. There are problems in using assessment in this way since the students can become too exam-oriented and lose sight of the real reason for learning (i.e. to provide the best possible quality of health care). This is particularly dangerous if the assessment is based solely on tests of knowledge.

However, where the assessment is related to the knowledge, attitudes and the whole range of skills involved in health care, frequent assessments can motivate both students and teachers to higher levels of effort.

There are some commonly mentioned reasons for assessing students which the authors regard as either *much less important or as positively harmful*. These are as follows.

(i) To Place Students in an Order of Merit

This is unnecessary as there is little point in being rated 4th rather than 5th best in a group. What does matter is the overall standard of performance achieved. It can also be harmful as students may compete against one another rather than helping each other to all achieve the highest standard possible. A further disadvantage of this approach is that the kind of assessment which places students in order effectively (called norm-referenced testing) tends to work best when the questions asked are about the details and the more obscure facts. So this type of assessment encourages students to learn the details rather than the more fundamental parts of the course.

(ii) To Use the Examinations as a Way of Keeping Control over Students

This approach is also harmful as it tends to create divisions between teacher and learner. Further, it should never be necessary.

Summing up the reasons for assessing students: assessment should take place during the learning process to motivate students and to guide both students and teachers about what has been learnt well and about what still needs to be learnt. Secondly, at the end of the learning process assessment should be used to certify whether a student has achieved a satisfactory standard of performance.

8.3 SOME CONSEQUENCES FOR ASSESSMENT

If the reasons for assessment given above are accepted, then a number of consequences follow. These are as follows.

(i) Assessment should be 'Criterion-referenced'

The phrase 'criterion-referenced' means that the pass standard for an examination should be based on some previously defined standard of performance. This is different from examinations where the pass standard is related to the standard of other students (called *norm-referenced*).

An example of a norm-referenced examination would be one where the best 50 students passed or where the best 70% of the students passed or where a prize is awarded to the best student. A criterion-referenced examination would be one where every student who could do say 95% of the tasks taught in the course would pass. (Notice that this might be all of the students or possibly none of the students—what would matter would be whether each student reached the criterion.)

Criterion-referenced examinations are desirable because the criterion should be related to an acceptable standard of health care. Items will be tested because they are an important part of health care. This type of examination is also desirable because it tends to encourage students to co-operate with each other.

(ii) Assessment should be Continuous

In some courses, the only time when students are assessed is at the end of the course. This is clearly too late to guide either students or teachers since students who do badly will have no opportunity to correct their weaknesses; poor teaching (shown by large numbers of students making similar mistakes) cannot be put right at this stage.

Therefore, there should be fairly frequent assessment throughout a course so that there is time left to remedy errors or weaknesses.

Frequent assessment will also provide regular motivation throughout a course. This is clearly preferable to the single end-of-course examination where students can sometimes not bother much for the first half or three-quarters of a course and then become over-anxious when they realise that the end-of-course examination is approaching.

Therefore the assessment should take place regularly through a course at fairly frequent intervals (frequent assessment would be a more accurate phrase than the more usual term of continuous assessment). This does not mean that there should be regular examinations; what is required is that students should be asked to perform health skills (and possibly asked questions about their health care knowledge) on a frequent and regular basis. This performance should be observed (by students, teachers or qualified health workers) and the quality of the performance judged. This judgement should be passed on to the learners and to the teachers.

(iii) Assessment should be Diagnostic

These frequent assessments should aim to provide guidance to the students about what still needs to be learnt, and to teachers about what still needs to be taught. Therefore there is little point in telling a student 'You scored 65% in that test'. This does not tell the student which parts were done well and where mistakes were made.

Therefore the assessment should be diagnostic. That is, it should diagnose where additional learning is needed.

To do this, the overall figure of 65% is useless. It is far better to say things like:

'Your knowledge of well construction is sufficient but you need to study the methods of ventilating pit latrines.'

or

'You have prescribed the correct treatment for this patient but you failed to explain to her how and when to take the tablets.'

This may sound rather laborious but can be done quite simply by handing back to students their own marked answer papers (for written assessments) or by using checklists (for practical assessments).

8.4 FEATURES OF EFFECTIVE ASSESSMENT

Assessment may be criterion-referenced, continuous and diagnostic, but it will still be a waste of time (or possibly harmful) unless the assessment has two features or characteristics. These are that the assessment should be both 'Valid' and 'Reliable'. What do these two technical words mean?

Valid Assessment

An assessment is *valid* if it actually measures what it is intended to measure. This rather general definition may be translated into more practical terms in the context of Primary Health Care (PHC) by saying that an assessment is valid if it actually measures whether a student can provide effective health care.

For example, a teacher might want to know whether the students are able to diagnose whether patients are anaemic or not. The most valid way to do this would be to observe each student in the normal working environment and ask the student to decide whether each of a number of patients was anaemic or not. This assessment matches almost exactly what the teacher wants to find out. It also tests whether the student can perform a task which is likely to be a part of their future work.

A much less valid assessment would be to ask the students to write an essay on 'How to diagnose anaemia'. This would be less valid because some people are better at writing about diagnosis than they are at actually doing it. On the other hand some people may be capable of diagnosing anaemia but are rather poor at writing. So the essay is related in some way to the actual skill to be tested, but is not by any means exactly the same thing.

An even less valid assessment would be to ask the students to 'Write short notes on anaemia'. This is further away from the actual skill to be assessed. In fact it asks the students to do something which they are most unlikely to ever have to do as a health worker. How often do patients come to a clinic and ask the health worker for 'some short notes on anaemia, please'?

The importance of assessment being valid is that non-valid assessments can:
- Certify students as fit to provide health care where they are not—or vice versa. (Many assessments are non-valid because they test

mainly knowledge rather than performance of health care skills. These tests can 'pass' students with a lot of book knowledge but little practical ability. These tests can also 'fail' students with the practical skill but weak ability to express their knowledge in written form.)
- Fail to provide useful guidance on what needs to be learnt, since non-valid assessments do not test what really needs to be learnt.
- Encourage students to learn things which are less important (e.g. how to write essays rather than how to talk with village people). So non-valid assessments will motivate students wrongly.

Assessment can, in principle, be made valid very simply. This is done by making the assessment item reflect precisely the task which students are being taught. For example, when the task is

'Advise mothers on the preparation of weaning foods'

then the assessment (in principle) should be to take each student to a clinic or a home and under the normal working conditions actually advise mothers on the preparation of weaning foods. In other words, the assessment should be based on observing the student perform each of the tasks defined in chapter 4.

In principle this is easy. In practice there are obviously formidable difficulties. The ways in which these very serious difficulties can be at least partially overcome will be explained in the chapters on Teaching and Assessing.

The crucial point here is that teachers should aim to make assessment as valid as possible—even though this will often be difficult.

Reliable Assessment

An assessment is *reliable* if it provides a consistent and accurate judgement of the competence of a student.

For example, suppose a teacher assessed a student and at the end of the assessment process said, 'This student is competent to provide health care'. Then another teacher assessed the same student and said. 'This student is *not* competent to provide health care'. The results of the assessment of this student are different and so the assessment process is not reliable.

Why might the teachers reach different verdicts? Some of the many reasons are:

- The student actually performed to a different standard in the two assessment procedures. (Students do vary in their performance depending on their state of health, their level of anxiety, the time of day, etc., etc.)
- The two teachers had different ideas about the standard of competence required.
- The two teachers asked the students to do different things—the first teacher asking things which the student was good at, the second teacher asking things where the student was not so good.

Where these possible causes of differences are eliminated or reduced, the assessment is made more reliable.

This can be done by:

- Assessing students on several different occasions (i.e. using frequent assessment) so that the variations in the students' performance will average out. This also has the advantage that the tension will be less and so the students' performance will be less affected by anxiety.
- Using an agreed marking scheme or a checklist, so that standards of performance can be better agreed. This also has the advantage that the marking scheme or checklist can be given to the students after the test so that they can see in detail what they need to learn.

    Differences of standards between different examiners can also be reduced by using multiple-choice questions instead of essays (see 'Teaching and Assessing Knowledge').

    Another technique is to use several examiners or markers and either averaging the marks they give or asking them to reach an agreed decision.
- Basing the overall result on the results of a large number of tests (e.g. instead of testing clinical competence using a 'long case' and a 'short case', test clinical competence by observing students on a large number of occasions when they are working with patients).

In these ways the assessment system can be made more *reliable*, that is, the assessment system will give a mark or a decision which reflects the true ability of each student.

8.5 SOME ISSUES IN ORGANISING ASSESSMENT

So far, the emphasis in this chapter has been on what one should aim for in planning the assessment for a course. There has been little discussion of what can be realistically achieved. So first some of the problems will be discussed and then the final section of the chapter will look at ways in which a realistic assessment scheme might work for an imaginary course.

Three of the most common and serious problems are as follows.

A. Balance of Time

It can sometimes seem that in order to assess each student thoroughly, validly and reliably, the teachers should spend so much time in assessing that there is no time left for anything else. This particular problem can sometimes be partly solved by using other health workers to do the assessing. But even so, the students must have time for learning. So where should the balance come?

Before answering the question, the distinction must be made between four different types of assessment.

One is the assessment which takes place during the teaching and whilst students are practising skills under supervision. During this time, the more that students are actively involved in making decisions, communicating and performing manual skills, the better. And, of course, the more that their performance is assessed and feedback given to students, the better. So this type of assessment should really be literally continuous; there cannot be too much of it.

The second type of assessment is the slightly more formal kind of observation whilst students are working in the field. This is normally done by health workers who are not full time teachers. Here the situation is slightly different. Students will need to have some time for practising health care skills without being observed all the time and the health workers will have other responsibilities. So it is probably reasonable to expect the health worker to be actually observing the student for some 10–30% of the time and basing reports on this observation.

The third type of assessment is sometimes called a practice examination or test. The essential features of this are that full feedback is given to the student on his performance and that the result does not count towards the overall result of the course. It is probably reasonable to spend about 10% of the course time in this kind of test.

The final type of assessment is the examination (either practical or written) which counts (with the reports of field work) towards the overall result. The correct amount of time for this type of assessment varies very much with the length of course and with the skills and knowledge to be learnt. Possibly about 2% (for a long course) up to 5% (for a shorter course) might be a reasonable amount of time to be allocated. This time should be distributed through the course so as not to create too much tension at the end.

B. Traditions

Assessment of PHC students is often modelled on the traditions of assessment in medical school or colleges of nursing. These traditions may not be especially helpful in these institutions; they are certainly unhelpful when one is assessing in PHC. This is because the qualities required of an effective PHC worker are quite different from the qualities required of a hospital doctor or nurse. So there is no reason to adopt traditional methods.

Examples of traditions which should be very seriously questioned include:

(i) The emphasis on written and oral examinations. PHC workers should be able to communicate with the community (which is not the same as talking to an examiner or writing an essay) and provide health care. This is what should be assessed directly.

(ii) The pass mark of 50%. This is a specially dangerous tradition. Originally it had some merit in examinations which were designed to identify the best students and put them in order of merit. But this is not the aim of assessment in PHC training. The aim is to set a criterion of competence and so 50% is clearly far too low. (If a health worker is only right 50% of the time, he or she is clearly very dangerous.) So, much higher pass marks should be used.

This means in turn that the testing should not be of obscure details, but of fundamental facts and regularly used skills.

C. Lack of Expertise

Designing an effective assessment scheme for a training programme requires just as much skill as performing a lumbar puncture or diagnosing the causes of a 'red eye'. Yet many teachers and examiners have little training in the specific skills involved. As a result, assessment schemes in training programmes are often unreliable or invalid. Whilst this book attempts to give some guidance on assessment methods, it can only serve as a preliminary guide. Most teachers would benefit from additional training in the specific techniques of assessment.

8.6 SOME ASSESSMENT METHODS

A table of assessment methods (table 8.1) which are appropriate in training PHC staff is given below. Inevitably the table is not complete and sometimes the names for the techniques may be different from the names used elsewhere. Despite these limitations the list gives a reminder of the range of techniques available and the type of ability which each technique can best be used for.

The methods of assessment are described in the relevant chapters. However, there is one technique which is very useful in assessing all kinds of skills. This is called the Objective Structured Practical Examination and is described below as it is relevant to all of the various types of knowledge and skill.

Table 8.1 Methods of assessment

Assessing knowledge (chapter 10)	*Assessing attitudes* (chapter 11)	*Assessing communication skills* (chapter 12)	*Assessing manual skill* (chapter 13)	*Assessing decision-making skill* (chapter 14)
MCQs Short-answer questions Oral Open book exam *but not* essay questions	Observation in the field (checklist) Rating scale, 11.12	Role play (checklist) Observation in field (checklist), 12.8 Project work, 12.9 *but not* oral exams	Observation in the field/lab/clinic (checklists), 13.6c Rating scales, 13.6c 'Procedure book', 13.6c	'Patient' management problems, 14.9 Observed field work, 14.13 and 14.14

All (except perhaps attitudes) can be assessed using the OSPE.

8.7 THE OBJECTIVE STRUCTURED PRACTICAL EXAMINATION (OSPE)

The OSPE is a way of organising tests of communication skills, manual skills, decision-making skills and knowledge. Indeed a well-designed OSPE would test the students' ability in all these areas.

The Overall Method

The main characteristic of the OSPE is that it consists of about 20 'stations'. Each student starts the examination at a different station. At the station the student answers a question which may be either practical or written. At the end of a fixed time period (usually 5 min) a bell rings and each student moves on to the next station. By the end of the examination every students has visited every station.

This main feature (which is rather like the 'spot' examinations sometimes used in anatomy) is only part of the idea of the OSPE. Another feature is that the stations usually come in pairs—a 'practical station' followed by a 'written station'. At the practical station the student may be asked to examine some part of a patient (a full examination is not possible in the 5 min), explain something to a patient, examine data or photographs (including X-rays or the results of laboratory tests), take a history, or use a piece of equipment (e.g. a sphygmomanometer or a microscope).

The written station will usually be a few multiple-choice or short-answer questions based on the task performed at the practical station.

A further feature of the OSPE is that the practical stations may be observed by an examiner who uses a checklist or rating scale to assess the student's performance. In a typical 20 station examination there may be between 3 and 6 observed stations.

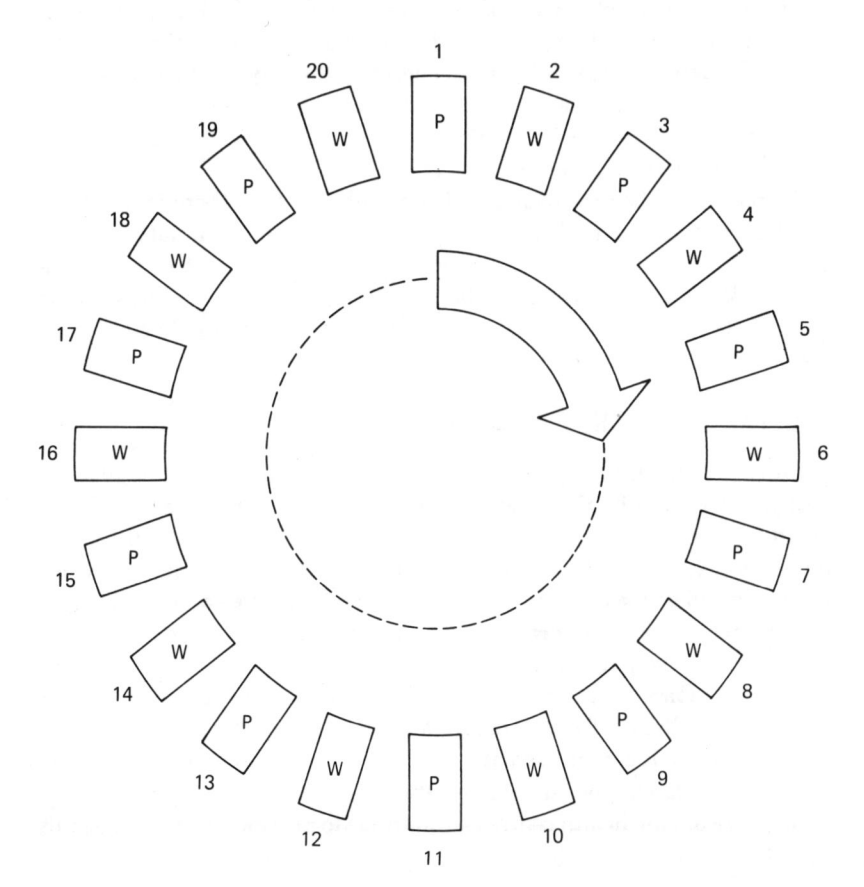

Figure 8.1 The OSPE

Why Bother to Use an OSPE?

From this brief description it must be obvious that organising an OSPE will take more effort than the simple essay-type examination. Although the organisational effort will become less with experience of running these exams, there must still be considerable benefits to justify the additional work.

In fact, the benefits are substantial.

Firstly, the examination is fair and is more reliable than other assessments of practical skills. The reason is that *all* students are asked to do the same tasks and to answer the same questions. Where practical assessment takes place in the field, students face different circumstances, different problems, different patients. They also face different examiners in the field whereas in the OSPE, each student has the same examiners. Moreover, the examiners are guided by checklists to help them mark to a more uniform standard.

Secondly, the examination is more reliable as it samples from quite a wide range of abilities and areas of the course. Remember that there are usually about 20 stations which gives more variety than in many practical or clinical examinations.

Thirdly, the OSPE is reasonably valid. A well designed OSPE will ask the student to do those things which they would normally do in the field as a qualified health worker. Therefore, the assessment tasks can be more or less the same as the objectives of the course, and so an OSPE can be valid. Another fact which increases validity is that the student is observed during the performance of the task. Therefore the way in which the task is performed can be assessed. This compares with some other practical assessments where the only thing which is assessed is the result or outcome of the practical work.

Despite these factors which indicate high validity, there is a serious restriction on the tasks which can be performed (i.e. they cannot take more than 5 min, or, exceptionally, 10 min). And, of course, the fact that the OSPE takes place under examination conditions inevitably reduces validity. Despite these qualifications, an OSPE can be substantially more valid than any written examination.

Where Can an OSPE Take Place?

Because an OSPE usually has about 20 stations, quite a lot of space is needed. Successful OSPEs have been organised in hospital wards, in health centres and in classrooms and lecture rooms. Naturally the use of these spaces will require co-operation from the people who normally use the space and so the benefits of OSPEs must be explained and possibly the service personnel or patients can be invited to help in the OSPE as 'examiners' or as 'patients'.

An ideal space would have several different rooms—or a large room which can be divided by screens. In many ways a health centre is the ideal place, provided it can be used at a time when there are comparatively few patients—as can happen during the afternoon.

In figure 8.2 the health centre can continue to provide a clinic and health

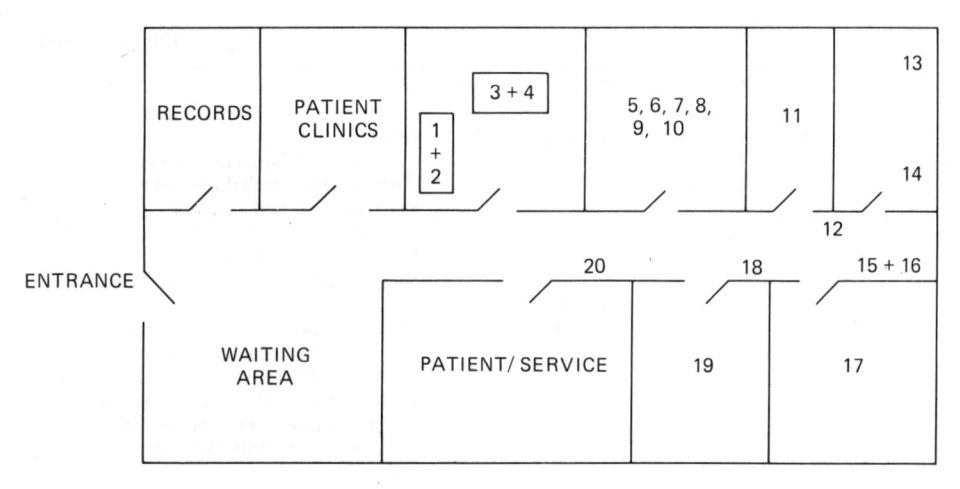

Figure 8.2 The use of a Health Centre for an OSPE

care service, whilst the examination takes over one end of the building. Stations 11, 17, 19 may involve talking to a patient and since the noise of this would be distracting, they take place in separate rooms (or a screened area of a ward). The questions following talking to a patient are written questions about the patient and so can be answered at a small table in the corridor. Stations 1 and 3 might involve some physical examination of a patient, so both can be in the same room (provided this causes no embarrassment to the patients) and the following 'written stations' (2 and 4) can also be in the same room. Stations 5 to 10 and 13, 14 may involve examination of a specimen, observation of photographs or data, etc., etc. Since these are all quiet stations they can be in the same room.

Some Examples of Stations

The questions or instructions for each student are written down on a piece of paper at each station. (It is wise to fasten the questions to the desk or the wall, so that students do not carry them away by mistake.) Some examples of questions or instructions are given in table 8.2.

Table 8.2

Question or Instruction	*Comment*
1. This patient complains of tiredness. You suspect anaemia. Carry out an examination to determine whether the patient appears to be anaemic. (N.B. No facilities for rapid blood tests are available.) Do not take a history	The 'patient' may be a real patient who is willing to be examined several times by different students. An alternative is to have a simulated patient. In each case the patient needs to look tired, but may or may not be anaemic. This station should be observed by an examiner, using a checklist, to assess the way in which the examination is carried out. The following written station could ask about the signs observed, the conclusion reached by the student, what the student would do next

Table 8.2 (contd)

Question or Instruction	Comment
2. This patient complains of a cough. Take a history. Do not examine the patient	Again the patient may be real or else simulated. The station should be observed to assess the manner in which the student communicates with the patient. The following written station can be used to establish what facts the student has obtained and what conclusions he comes to
3. Measure the blood pressure of this patient	This is another station where an examiner should observe the method used by the student. The following station could ask the student what blood pressure was observed. Additional questions might be of the type: What would you do if a 50-yr-old patient had a BP of 150/100?
4. This woman has come to the clinic for a check-up after giving birth 5 weeks ago. You have found that she and the baby are both well. Now try to persuade her to use some form of contraception. (N.B. The wording and the task itself should vary according to the health policy in different countries)	This patient should be 'simulated'. Ideally the 'patient' will not be a health worker but will have had a very brief training session to discuss the kind of responses she should make. This station should be observed to assess the way in which the student communicates
5. Look at this photograph of a village to identify any probable hazards to health. (A photograph of a local village is supplied)	No need for an examiner to observe. Following written station can ask what hazards have been seen, and possibly what can be done about one or two of them
6. Focus and adjust the light source of this microscope. Then look at the slide. (The need to focus and/or adjust light sources may be deleted if this would take too much time)	This does not need observation. It will need an assistant to put the microscope out of adjustment after each student. The following written station can ask specific questions about what was seen on the slide
7. This woman has brought her child to be immunised. A DPT injection has been given. Now explain why she must come back for a second and third injection	This station should be observed to assess the manner of the communication. The observer could be the 'mother' who completes a checklist at the end of the 5 min. This is an ideal station for a simulated patient

The above examples are intended simply to illustrate the possibilities and to show how stations can be organised as pairs of practical and written stations. Clearly the tasks must be adapted to suit the type of health worker being trained and the local conditions.

Some Issues Raised by OSPEs

One of the commonest difficulties in organising OSPEs is the repeated examination of a patient by possibly twenty students. This inevitably limits the kind of examination which can be performed, and the kind of patient on whom it can be performed.

The problem can be tackled in two ways. One is to have substitute patients with similar medical conditions. One patient is then examined by the first five students and then has a rest whilst the other patient is examined by the next five, and so on.

The other approach is to use simulated patients. Naturally a simulated patient cannot simulate wounds, enlarged spleens or dilated pupils. But simulated patients can learn a medical history and can simulate pain and quite a range of symptoms. It is surprisingly easy to train simulated patients in quite a short time to give a very convincing performance—especially where this mainly involves communication rather than physical examination. The best people to train as simulated patients are *not* health workers, but other members of the public. Relatives of teachers, secretaries, members of theatre groups and former patients have all been successfully used.

Another issue is that the OSPE is inevitably rather hectic and students must be limited to 5 min or so at each station (in order to complete enough stations in a short time). So it is not possible to test students' skills in performing longer tasks (such as attending a village health committee meeting, or conducting an examination of shop premises). Therefore an OSPE should only be a part of the whole assessment scheme.

Despite this limitation, there are many tasks or parts of tasks which health workers do have to complete in a restricted amount of time. Indeed one of the problems of training is that sometimes it ignores the very serious time limitations which health workers face in the field.

Preparing for an OSPE

Because an OSPE is a little different from more traditional examinations, it is vital that both teachers and students prepare for the examination. It is very strongly recommended that practice examinations are attempted before OSPEs are used to assess whether students pass or fail. This is *not* a waste of time. In fact one of the greatest values of the OSPE is as a learning experience. It is an excellent way of rounding off a section of a course, since it can test a range of skills quickly and detailed feedback (from the observers' checklists) can be given to the students.

The stages in organising the OSPE are:

(1) Write the instructions or questions which will appear at each station.
(2) Plan where in the examination space each of the stations will be placed. (Take into account whether the station will be noisy or quiet, whether it will need electricity, light, water, or a sink.) Remember that written stations will have to come immediately after their corresponding practical station. Aim to have the students progressing in a circle as much as possible so as to reduce walking between stations.
(3) Prepare an answer sheet—which each student carries round the examination with him. This must have sufficient space for the student to answer every question, but will not have the questions printed on it. An example is given below.

```
                    Answer Sheet
Name of student .............................    Date ...............

                    Starting station ........

Station 2      Circle the correct response
    Q. 1         A     B     C     D     E
    Q. 2         A     B     C     D     E
    Q. 3         A     B     C     D     E

Station 4
    Q. 1 ................................................
         ................................................
    Q. 2 ................................................
         ................................................
```

Note that the student does not answer a question at stations 1 or 3 as these are practical stations. The questions at station 2 are multiple choice whilst at station 4 they are short answers.

Providing an answer sheet makes the whole process of marking very much easier.

(4) Prepare a checklist for each station where there is an observer or examiner. Train the observer how to use the checklist. (Note that senior students, secretaries, junior teachers, service personnel and simulated patients have all been used successfully as examiner/observers.)
(5) Train any simulated patients.
(6) Make sure any needed equipment is available and in the right place.
(7) Make sure that a bell and clock is available to signal when students should move from one station to the next.
(8) Prepare a master mark sheet to record student marks, as shown.

Student Name	MASTER MARK SHEET																				
	1	2	3	4	5	6	7	8	9	10	11	12	13	14	15	16	17	18	19	20	Total
1.																					
2.																					
3.																					
4.																					
5.																					
6.																					
7.																					

Note that this allows teachers to see very quickly which stations have resulted in high marks and where the marks are low. This gives good feedback to teachers about where additional or improved teaching is needed.

(9) Decide where each student is to start the examination—this can be written on the Answer Sheet.

When deciding on starting stations, one should note that it is *not* possible to start at a written station if the written answer depends on information obtained at the previous practical station. So assume station 15 is a written station which depends on station 14. One student will have to be told 'go to station 15 but do not attempt to answer the question there. Wait until the bell goes and then move on to station 16'. The question at station 15 should be covered up so the student cannot read it. Then the cover should be removed at the first bell.

This outline of the preparation for the examination will need to be adapted to suit local conditions, but covers the main points. A more detailed description of the OSPE technique with a very full checklist appears in the ASME Booklet No. 8 by R. M. Harden and F. A. Gleeson. This is available from the Association for the Study of Medical Education, Roseangle, Dundee, Scotland.

OSPE with a Large Number of Students

The most convenient situation is when a 20 station OSPE is organised for 20 students. If there are fewer students, then some of the stations will not be occupied at any one time. This is not a problem—and in fact gives patients and observers a break, so is a good thing.

When there are more than 20 students then they should be divided into two groups. The OSPE can then be run twice with a half hour break in between. The two groups of students can easily be kept apart during this break.

If there are more than 40 students, two OSPEs with similar patients can take place at the same time. 120 medical students have been assessed in one morning using three simultaneous OSPEs followed immediately by another three. This does require substantial organisation and resources, but is quite possible.

OSPE Summary

The technique combines well established features of other methods of examining. It is initially difficult to organise and practice examinations are essential. However, the effort is well worth while in achieving a reliable and fairly valid assessment of a wide range of communication, decision-making and manual skills. The technique, adapted to suit local conditions, can provide a very valuable part of the overall assessment scheme.

SUMMARY

- Assessment should be used frequently to guide the students about what needs to be learnt and to help the learning process.
- Assessments should also be made about whether students should be certified to provide health care. This type of assessment should concentrate on the skill of the student to perform the common skills involved in health care. A high pass mark should be required.
- Effective assessment is both *valid* and *reliable*.
- The method of assessment chosen should match the type of ability being assessed (see table 8.1).
- An example of how assessment methods could be organised in a specific course is provided in Appendix 4.

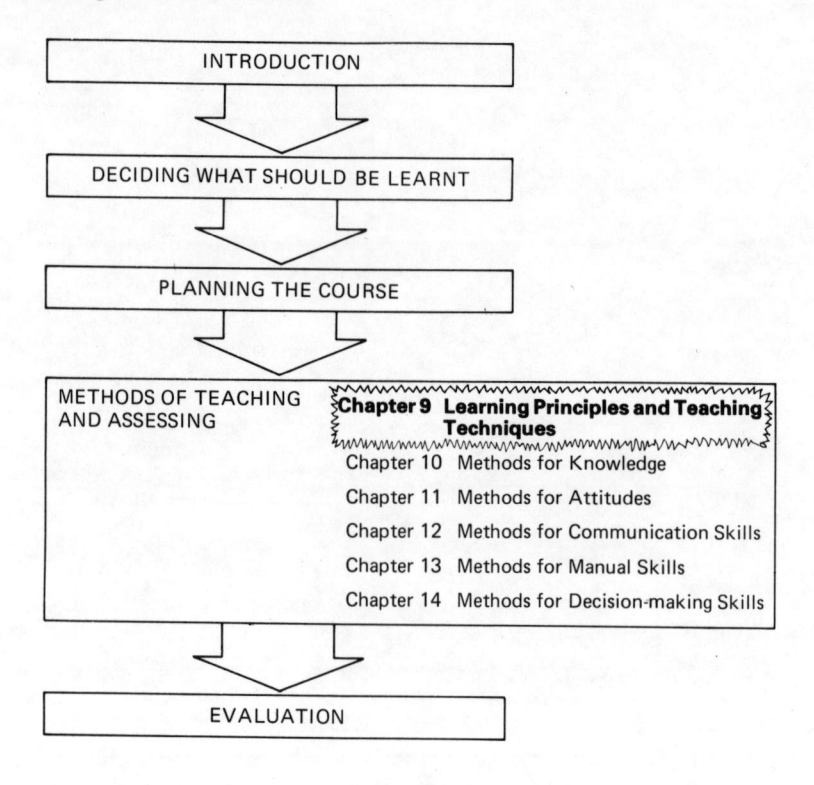

```
        INTRODUCTION
             ↓
  DECIDING WHAT SHOULD BE LEARNT
             ↓
      PLANNING THE COURSE
             ↓
┌─────────────────────┬──────────────────────────────────────┐
│ METHODS OF TEACHING │ Chapter 9  Learning Principles and   │
│ AND ASSESSING       │            Teaching Techniques       │
│                     │ Chapter 10 Methods for Knowledge     │
│                     │ Chapter 11 Methods for Attitudes     │
│                     │ Chapter 12 Methods for Communication │
│                     │            Skills                    │
│                     │ Chapter 13 Methods for Manual Skills │
│                     │ Chapter 14 Methods for Decision-     │
│                     │            making Skills             │
└─────────────────────┴──────────────────────────────────────┘
             ↓
         EVALUATION
```

CONTENTS

9.1	Learning Principles	105
9.2	Wanting to Learn—Motivation	105
9.3	Social Relationships	107
9.4	Physical Environment	107
9.5	Clarity	108
9.6	Relevance to the Future	109
9.7	Relevance to Previous Experience	109
9.8	Structure	110
9.9	Active Learning	112
9.10	Feedback	113
9.11	Speed	113
9.12	Some Methods for Improving Clarity and Structure	114
9.13	Handouts and Manuals	115
9.14	Some Methods for Encouraging Active Participation	115

9
Learning Principles and Teaching Techniques

In previous chapters the question of 'What should be learnt?' has been considered. Once this has been decided, teachers are likely to ask 'What is the best way of teaching this part of the course?'

To anwer this question, the ways in which students learn must be understood. Then this understanding should be applied to the learning objectives so as to work out exactly what the teacher can do to help learning.

This chapter will first of all explain some of the ways in which students learn, that is, the Learning Principles. Then a number of more frequently used teaching techniques will be described.

9.1 LEARNING PRINCIPLES

The principles of learning are not based on an exact science like physics where the laws of physics allow one to predict very precisely how a beam of light will pass through a lens or a transistor will react to electric currents. On the other hand, teaching is not just an art. Effective teaching is based on principles. The principles do not state exactly how much will be learnt under different circumstances, instead they indicate which methods are *likely* to be more helpful. These principles have become established as a result of extensive research and experience. Yet they are still subject to debate, with some teachers arguing about whether one principle is more important than another.

So what follows is a very brief summary of some of the principles which have become established. Applying these principles will make it *more likely* (though not certain) that students will learn. Applying the principles will also help students to learn faster and more permanently.

It is important therefore for teachers to understand these principles and apply them to the courses which they teach.

9.2 WANTING TO LEARN—MOTIVATION

> Students learn faster and more thoroughly when they want to learn

This is both entirely obvious and very important. The difficulty for the teacher is to create the conditions in which the students will want to learn.

The first point to make is that it is natural for people to want to learn. Learning, just like eating or sleeping, is a basic function of human beings. Consider how rapidly babies and young children learn, as they explore the environment and learn to speak their mother tongue. People go on learning all their lives. But adults are more selective in their learning than young children. Young children explore most things that come their way, adults learn things which are useful to them or which interest them.

Naturally some people are more eager to learn than other people—in the same way that some people tend to be hungrier for food than other people. This internal eagerness to learn is part of the student's personality and cannot be changed much by the teacher. It is sometimes called the student's 'level of motivation'. However, it is a mistake for teachers who are faced with a specially dull and uninterested group of students to assume that they all have a low level of motivation. A much more likely explanation is that the students have varying levels of motivation within themselves—but they have had discouraging experiences which make them seem less motivated.

What can teachers do to help students want to learn? All of the principles outlined below will help students to become more motivated. For example, relating learning to the future job will make the learning seem much more worth while and so tend to increase motivation. On the other hand failing to apply the principles will tend to discourage the student and reduce his motivation. (For example, if the teacher persistently uses long and unfamiliar words, the student will not be able to understand and so cannot be interested in what is being said.)

There are other more specific actions which teachers can take which affect motivation. When students produce good work or show that they have learnt, the teacher should praise or encourage the student and in this way *reward* the learning. This will tend to increase motivation. On the other hand, failure to reward or persistent and possibly unfair criticism will usually decrease motivation.

Another method is to create some tension or anxiety in the students. For example, if the students are told that they will have a test of their skill, then this creates some tension or anxiety. The consequence is that the students are likely to learn faster. However, if too much tension is created then this

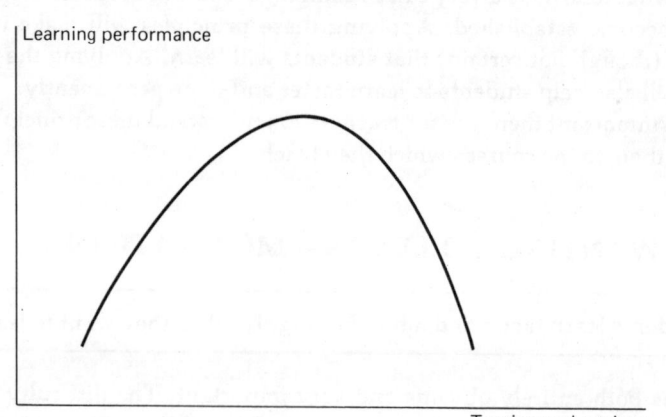

Figure 9.1 The relationship between learning performance and level of tension and anxiety

will interfere with learning and so will be counter productive. The 'ideal' amount of tension varies from one person to another and so teachers must be very sensitive to the effects which any attempt to increase anxiety actually has. Techniques which increase tension are any forms of tests or examinations or competition. Many students will also experience anxiety when using a technique with real patients for the first time or as the deadline for handing in a project approaches.

Teachers may not wish to deliberately introduce additional tensions or anxieties into the learning situation. However, they should be aware of the effects which are likely to result from the various causes of tension and anxiety which are inevitably present.

9.3 SOCIAL RELATIONSHIPS

> Learning is affected by the social relationships between the people involved

Learning usually takes place in a group setting. The relationship between the teacher and the learners can be an important negative or positive influence. Also the relationship between the different learners is influential. These relationships combine together to provide an atmosphere or mood in the learning situation.

Most PHC students are adults. They respond best to an atmosphere of acceptance, respect and encouragement. Students should feel free to ask questions and contribute to class discussion. They will not do so if the teacher humiliates them or makes them look foolish in front of their fellow students. Nor will they be at ease if the teacher shows favouritism towards some class members.

Creating an atmosphere where individuals feel able to work, learn and contribute depends on the teacher developing an attitude of respect for his students. This attitude will be taken up by the students who will learn to respect each other.

Having respect for the students is essential. But teachers can also arrange matters so that the social relationships can develop. At the beginning of a course time should be spent in letting students get to know each other and the teachers. Maybe there should be some parties. Certainly there should be a lot of sessions in which students and teachers will discuss and will solve problems as a team. This pattern will allow the social relationships to develop. Starting a course with a full timetable of lectures will almost certainly prevent the development of the very important group confidence.

9.4 PHYSICAL ENVIRONMENT

> The physical surrounding can also affect learning. The basic principle is that learning takes place best when there are no distractions

The physical environment should be quiet and at a comfortable temperature. Poor ventilation or overcrowding will decrease the rate of learning.

An ideal room for a group of 20–25 students should have a floor area of 60–80 m² and be approximately square. There should be good ventilation and sufficient light from the windows. There should be some form of chalkboard and ideally a screen for a projector. (If there is a projector then it should be possible to darken the room without stopping the ventilation.) It should ideally be possible to control the temperature, but in any case the temperature should be reasonably comfortable for the students. The furniture should include moveable desks and chairs so that students can face each other during discussion or face the screen/chalkboard when material is presented there.

9.5 CLARITY

> For students to learn, the messages communicated to the students must be clear

This principle is a very obvious one, but can be difficult to put into practice. The clarity will depend on:

(i) *The words and sentence structures used.* The words should be familiar to the students. When new technical words are introduced, they should be explained and the students' understanding checked. Sentences should be short and should not use many clauses. Pronouns (words like 'it', 'they', 'this') should only be used rarely.

(ii) *Messages should be visual.* Most people can learn more quickly and permanently by looking rather than by hearing. So, at the lowest level, the students should be allowed to read as well as to hear (provided that the students are literate). The message will have more impact if it is in a visual/pictorial form than if it is just words. So diagrams, pictures and models should be used where possible.

Whichever type of visual aid is used, certain rules make them more effective.

- They must be visible to the whole class. This may seem obvious—but walk into any classroom and look at the small size or rough writing left on the blackboard! This obvious rule is unfortunately forgotten too often.
- Visual aids should be clear. Again, observation of blackboards will show the most extraordinary scrawls and squiggles and rough incomplete diagrams. When a student is unfamiliar with a topic, these displays bring confusion rather than clarity. (To overcome this problem, see Blackboard/Flip charts and OHPs.) Simplicity goes with clarity. Do not overcrowd.
- Diagrams should be simple and extract the essential elements. Complex diagrams are confusing and not helpful in the classroom. When a complex diagram is needed it should be given in a handout or referred to in a manual, where the student can study it at leisure.

- Visual aids must be relevant to the subject matter. This again is obvious—but some teachers show excess pictures in an effort to 'be visual'. Too many pictures are as confusing as too much talk.
- It is very important that any visual aid shown should coincide with the words being used. If a picture or a diagram is still visible when the teacher moves on to the next topic, the audience will have some of their attention still fixed on the picture. Each visual aid should be removed when the discussion to which it relates has ceased. Looking at one thing and hearing about something else is not the best way to learn!

9.6 RELEVANCE TO THE FUTURE

> In general, students will learn more rapidly when they realise that what they are learning will be useful to themselves in the future

In training for Primary Health Care (PHC), teachers can only assume that the students will want to be effective as PHC workers. So the courses must be very specifically related to the work which the students will be doing in the future. This is guaranteed if the choice of what the students learn is governed by the processes described in chapters 3–6.

However there is a difference between the course being relevant and the student realising that it is relevant. For learning to be fast, students must recognise the relevance of what they are learning.

Teachers can help students to recognise relevance by:

(i) Telling the students how each session will be useful in their future work.
(ii) Arranging for students to do work in the field as 'apprentice' PHC workers, so that the students themselves can see what they need to learn.

9.7 RELEVANCE TO PREVIOUS EXPERIENCE

> People learn faster when the new information or skill is related to what they already know or can do

New information will be learnt more quickly if it can be fitted into the structure of what is already known. For example, if one already knows the principles and techniques used in DPT immunisations, then one can learn about measles immunisation more quickly.

This benefit is only achieved when the relationship (i.e. the similarities and the differences) between what is already known and what is to be learnt are made clear. So one of the functions of the teacher is to:

(i) find out what learner(s) already know(s) and then
(ii) make the connections between the existing knowledge and the new.

Some teachers make the mistake of thinking that their students know very little. Yet these students will have a lot of experience of disease (either through being ill themselves or through knowing relatives or friends who have been ill) and of the cultural setting in which disease occurs. So, often a major part of the teaching is not so much giving new information, but drawing out, organising and building on what the learners already know.

Sometimes teachers must provide the experience, because students have previously had no opportunity. One example is the idea of very small organisms which students cannot have seen in their earlier experience. So in this case it seems essential to arrange for students to use magnifying glasses and then microscopes so that they can see these organisms for themselves. After this experience, diagrams and pictures will have much more meaning.

9.8 STRUCTURE

> Learning will be more rapid when the information or skills are presented in a structured way

Exercise

Look for about two or three seconds at the two diagrams in figure 9.2.

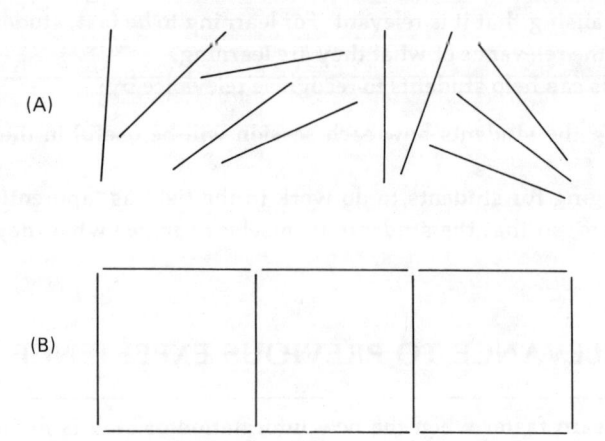

Figure 9.2

Now turn over the book and try to draw the diagrams A and B. When you have done this read on.

Comments on the Exercise

Almost certainly you could draw diagram B. It has a pattern to it which makes sense—three squares joined together. Diagram A was probably much more difficult to remember. There is no shape or meaning to it. But the number of lines in each case was exactly the same.

By 'structuring' knowledge we mean grouping information so that similar topics are learned together, systematising information so that it follows a pattern and arranging information in a sequence which follows a logical train of thought.

Why is this important? Information which is scattered about or which is muddled is much more difficult to understand and remember than information which is grouped, arranged and classified.

A teacher can demonstrate this for himself by playing the 'memory game' with his students (see below).

The Memory Game

Part 1

Place 18 objects on a large tray, 6 objects from each of 3 groups of articles (for example, eating utensils, foods, office materials)
Place the objects in a mixed up order and cover the tray with a cloth
In the classroom call 10 students to stand around the tray
Remove the cover and allow them to look for 1 minute
Cover the objects again
Ask the students to write down as many as they can remember

Part 2

Rearrange the tray outside the classroom
Arrange the objects into groups on the tray
   1. Eating utensils (e.g. plate, mug, glass, spoon, knife, fork)
   2. Foods (e.g. tomato, orange, tea, sugar, oil, beans)
   3. Office materials (e.g. pen, pencil, paper, envelope, rubber, paper clip)
Cover the tray
Call 10 different students, uncover and allow them to look for 1 minute—exactly the same as the first group
Cover the objects again
Ask the students to write down as many objects as they can remember

Now compare the answers of the two students groups
You will find that the second group remembered many more objects

---

How can a teacher help learning by 'structuring' information? He does this

- in curriculum design;
- in course programmes;
- in lesson-plans;
- in handouts and manuals.

(i) Curriculum Design

In arranging a curriculum topics are grouped together in some way. There are several ways to do this in health topics. For example, a course in 'clinical care' might be arranged under body systems—respiratory system, cardiovascular system, digestive system and so on; or it might be arranged under presenting symptoms—such as cough, diarrhoea, fever, skin rashes and so on. The way a curriculum is designed determines the way students will think about the topics and the way the information will be stored and used in their heads.

(ii) Course Programmes

A 'course' is one section of a curriculum—usually taught by one teacher.

When the teacher has decided the Task List for the course he will need to sequence it so that the parts follow in logical order. For example, in a course on nutrition it would be more 'logical' to study the constituents of various foods before discussing their effects within the body.

(iii) Lesson Plans

In planning lessons, teachers need to refer to what students already know and what they have previously learned. This helps the student to structure the information in his mind, connecting it with previous parts of the course. Also, the order in which the lesson is presented is likely to be the order in which it is remembered (see chapter 7, Planning a Lesson)

(iv) Handouts and Manuals

Most literate students study and learn from their handouts and manuals. If these are structured in a similar way to the course programme and the lessons, it will reinforce the students' learning. A handout or manual structured differently from the lessons can cause great confusion to students.

9.9 ACTIVE LEARNING

> Learning takes place quicker when students actively process information, solve problems or practise skills

Unfortunately for both teachers and students, simply presenting information, however perfectly done, does not in itself achieve learning.

Learning requires an active mental effort from the learner. This might take the form of recalling what has been learned or using the information in an exercise. Applying what is learned in a practical task or in a simulation or in a game are other ways of achieving active learning.

This is perhaps the most important learning principle and should be applied throughout all teaching. Sadly it is also the principle which seems to be least well applied in many training programmes.

Rather than listing here what teachers can do, some of the techniques which encourage active learning are briefly described at the end of this chapter and described in more detail throughout chapters 10–14.

9.10 FEEDBACK

When information is actively recalled or used by the student he needs to be sure that he is recalling it or using it correctly. Or if he has 'got it wrong' he needs to know that as soon as possible, before he continues 'learning the wrong thing'. The process by which a teacher informs a student that he is right or wrong is called *feedback*.

> Feedback increases the speed of learning

One way of understanding feedback is to think about a person learning to ride a bicycle. When he balances his body in a certain way he falls off. This tells him immediately that he has got the balance wrong. When he balances his body and moves correctly he stays on, then his body knows immediately that he has got it right. After repeated trial and error, through this feedback, he quickly learns to feel the right way of balancing to stay on the bicycle.

Teachers give feedback to students in many ways.

They give feedback when they comment on the quality of students' answers to questions, when they observe students doing health care tasks and advise the students about what is being done well and what is being done badly.

Feedback is most helpful when:

- it is immediate, i.e. straight after the student does something. Marking a project 2 weeks after it has been given in, is not immediate feedback;
- it states the standard of the performance, i.e. lists what is done well and what is done badly;
- it guides improvement, i.e. it explains how the performance can be improved or reach a higher standard.

Feedback is important when learning factual information or decision-making skills. It is provided when teachers comment on students' answers or solutions to problems.

9.11 SPEED

> Learning is fastest when the speed of presenting information matches the speed at which students can learn

Students learn at different speeds and this principle presents a serious problem to a teacher of a mixed class. If he goes too fast the slow students will get left behind, if he goes too slowly the fast students will become bored. Using the target concept (see page 126), and giving time for individual study, are two ways around this problem.

9.12 SOME METHODS FOR IMPROVING CLARITY AND STRUCTURE

Nearly every technique of teaching can, when it is used well, embody most of the Learning Principles outlined in the previous sections. Equally, no general technique guarantees that the Learning Principles will be followed. Nearly everything depends on how well the teacher uses the technique which he or she chooses.

With the qualification above, some techniques are designed to help the teacher put into practice some of the principles. In particular the range of techniques and equipment sometimes called *visual aids* specially help teachers to make their teaching clearer and better structured.

The visual aids which are commonly used include the following.

(i) Chalkboard, Flip Chart and Overhead Projector

These three instruments are all used for the same purpose—as visual aids in the classroom to display pictures, words, headings, notes and diagrams during a lesson.

Many teachers experience difficulty because they say they 'cannot draw'. There are several ways of overcoming this problem.

- Ask a student who can draw, to copy a picture or diagram onto a large sheet of newsprint or brown paper and stick this onto the wall.
- Trace pictures from books onto a stencil and give this to students as handouts. Trace pictures onto the Overhead Projector transparency.
- Project transparent slides onto a paper on the wall, and then trace the outline.
- Draw a diagram very carefully onto the blackboard before the class begins. Or ask a student to copy a diagram from a book onto the blackboard.

The chalkboard or blackboard and the OHP are also described in section 10.7.

(ii) Films and Slides and Other Visual Materials

A slide projector is a useful adjunct in the classroom, because a photograph comes nearer to reality than a diagram.

If a teacher has his own camera, he can show students the actual health situations in which they will be working. Alternatively, a wide range of slides, especially related to health care in the developing world is available from TALC (see Appendix 1).

Films are less often useful than slides. It is often difficult to find a film which is relevant to learning PHC. But where locally made documentary films on health care are available, they can be very powerful learning aids.

Posters are often available free from drug firms and international agencies. If a poster is left on the wall for too long it ceases to have impact. Posters need to be constantly changed so that they will be observed.

Photographs of village situations or health conditions can be handed around the class during a lesson.

Models are valuable aids. Models of the human body, skeleton, eye, ear and so on are available on request from UNICEF. Teachers can also make their own models from local materials.

(iii) Demonstrations

A demonstration is a lesson in which the visual aid approaches as nearly as possible to reality. How to conduct a demonstration is discussed in section 13.4.

9.13 HANDOUTS AND MANUALS

These are materials which help to structure learning and serve as reference material.

The way in which the material is structured and laid out is very important for learning.

A clear layout means that the structure of the learning becomes visible. The structure is the framework in which the knowledge is stored. Teachers need to take care with the layout of their handouts.

Handouts and manuals are discussed in chapter 10 (sections 10.7 and 10.5 respectively).

9.14 SOME METHODS FOR ENCOURAGING ACTIVE PARTICIPATION

(i) Using Discussion Methods

What are the Advantages of Discussions in the Classroom?

Discussion ensures a two-way dialogue between teacher and students.

It is a way of helping all or most students to actively contribute to the learning process. It is a quick way for a class to review their experiences and thus reinforce what has been learnt. It is a rapid way of finding out what a class has understood or remembered and of giving immediate feedback to confirm ideas or correct errors. It can be used to develop attitudes and also to encourage students to give expression to their ideas. It makes learning more active and more meaningful.

The Methods and their Use

Question and answer is used in many circumstances. At the introduction to a lesson to find out what students already know, where a teacher wishes to review what students have learned from an experience or a field visit, as an informal revision of knowledge or to lead into a discussion or a controversial issue.

Class discussion can be used at difficult points in a lesson or at the end of a topic for review purposes.

Syndicate discussion. In this the class is divided into several groups. Each group prepares a different assignment and reports back to the class. This is an interesting way of covering a wide area and is particularly useful when students do community surveys.

Debates and panels can be used to train students into thinking clearly about controversial topics. Debates need to be carefully controlled by the teacher to make sure the arguments are based on facts. In a Panel discussion several students prepare a topic and present it to the class, who then ask the panel questions.

Snowball discussion is a method of getting every single person involved in the discussion. The question or topic is posed by the teacher. Then it is discussed, first in pairs, then pairs join to make groups of four, then these join to make groups of eight. In this way each individual participates and each one hears many points of view expressed. This method is sometimes called the Pyramidal Group Method—because people join together like an inverted pyramid (Figure 9.3). The snowball method can also be used with written exercises (see section 14.8).

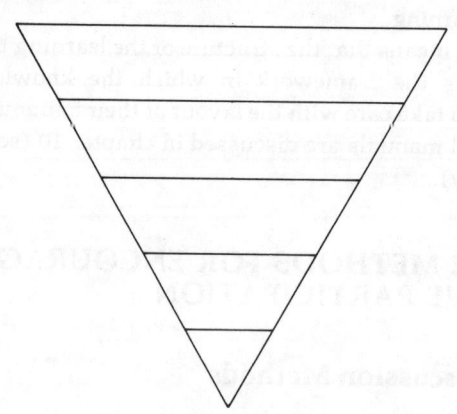

Figure 9.3

Brainstorm. This is a method of collecting ideas from individual members of a group on how to solve a problem. Ideas are given at great speed, and written down without criticism. When all the ideas have been collected, they are then reviewed by this group one at a time (see section 14.7).

(ii) Using Games

What are the Advantages of Using Games in Learning?

Games have recently become very popular in PHC training. They not only make learning enjoyable, but as they are enjoyed they get repeated and this reinforces learning. Games may be played by students outside class hours and so encourage self-study.

The Methods and their Use

Role play is used to illustrate situations or health problems which are complex and usually involved with certain community beliefs or values. They are used to reveal the essence of a situation and thus to develop attitudes towards the problem and its solution. A role play must have a clear objective and needs careful planning. After the role play the teacher guides the discussion to emphasise the main aspects learned. Students enjoy participating in a role play but without guidance from the teacher may lose sight of the intended message (see section 14.12).

Board and paper games. Several games on health topics have now been invented. Most of these games involve moving counters across a board after throwing dice. At intervals around the board certain health questions have to be answered correctly before proceeding. The student who knows the answers will reach the goal quickest. In this way, knowledge is absorbed while playing the game (see section 14.11).

Simulation games. These are games which involve complex situations in community health, for example, how to allocate a budget for a certain area, or how to make a health plan to solve certain problems. Participants are given an amount of demographic, geographic and health data and then asked to solve a particular problem. Sometimes the groups are asked to solve the problem in particular roles—such as the politician, the bureaucrat, the agitator and so on. In this case there is a combination of simulation and role play (see section 14.11).

(iii) Using Written Exercises

What are the Advantages of Written Exercises?

Written exercises encourage the student to actively recall, to think, to work out problems and to make decisions. Written exercises can be used in the classroom and for self-study.

The Methods and their Use

Written tests. Short written tests at the beginning or end of class sessions can be used to recall introductory material or as a method of summarising the main points of a lesson. To save teacher time, they should be corrected in class, by the students—and they then have the additional merit of acting as an immediate feedback.

Simulated written exercises. Because it is difficult to find enough real experience in health care, real situations can be described in writing and students can be asked to respond to questions related to the situation.

The usual examples of this technique are Patient Management Problems (PMP). In this exercise the patient's history and signs are presented step-by-step and the student is asked about his decisions as the case progresses (see section 14.9).

Group projects. Small groups of students may be given written assignments. They might have to do a survey, research into some literature or present some patient's clinical history to the class.

(iv) Using Self-study Activities

What are the Advantages of Self-study Activities?

All students have to study on their own, to absorb the learning which is presented to them. Usually, they are left without guidance and they sit and read their notes. This is not the best way to study because it is inactive and produces boredom and sleep!

If students are given guidelines for their private study, they are likely to progress faster. Active participation and involvement in learning is as important in private study as it is in the classroom.

The Methods and their Use

Peer learning. Students should be encouraged to work in pairs during their study periods, to ask each other questions or do assignments together.

Programmed learning. In this the student does exercises using a specially prepared book or tape, which proceeds by short steps and ask questions or sets problems at each stage. Only when one step is mastered can the student proceed to the next step. This is a very good way of learning. Unfortunately, setting up the programme is very time-consuming.

Individual project work. Students are given projects or assignments in which they must actively search for information.

Practical work. Most practical work is a form of self-study. Guidelines for this might be record books, procedure lists and checklists. These methods are discussed in chapter 13.

SUMMARY

Some important principles of learning are:

- wanting to learn;
- good relationships between teacher and students;
- good presentation, which is clear, relevant, meaningful well-structured and at the right speed;
- learning by active participation, supported by immediate feedback.

Teaching techniques are methods by which these principles are put into practice.

Some visual aids are:

- chalkboard, flipcharts, overhead projector;
- films and slides;
- posters, photographs;
- models;
- demonstrations;
- handouts and manuals.

Some ways of encouraging active learning are by:

- discussion methods;
- games;
- written exercises;
- self-study activities.

A list of techniques and their chapter references follows.

SOME TEACHING METHODS AND WHERE THEY ARE DESCRIBED

Straightforward lecturing, or the teacher talking in a classroom, is inevitably an inefficient way of teaching. Some of the alternatives are listed in table 9.1 together with a reference to the section where they are described.

Table 9.1

Methods	When they are especially useful*					Reference (section)	
	K	A	D	M	C		
Chalkboard	✓					9.12	10.7
OHP	✓					9.12	10.7
Slides/photographs	✓					9.12	10.7
Films	✓			✓	✓	9.12	
Handouts	✓		✓	✓		9.12	
Self-study	✓					9.13	10.7
Demonstrations				✓	✓	9.12	13.4
Manuals	✓		✓	✓	✓	9.12	10.5
Discussion		✓	✓		✓	9.13	
Brain-storming			✓		✓	14.7	
Snowballing		✓	✓			14.8	
Games	✓	✓	✓		✓	14.11	
Case studies			✓			14.9	
Flow charts	✓		✓			14.10	
Role play		✓	✓		✓	12.7	14.12
Written exercises plus project work	✓		✓		✓	12.9	
Observed field work		✓	✓	✓	✓	14.13	
Supervised field work		✓	✓	✓	✓	14.14	
Simulation			✓	✓	✓	13.4	
Paired practice				✓	✓	13.5c	
Procedure book				✓		13.6c	
Checklists				✓	✓	13.6c	
Rating scales				✓	✓	13.6c	
Roster				✓		13.6f	

* K = knowledge; A = attitudes; D = decision-making skills; M = manual skills; C = communication skills.

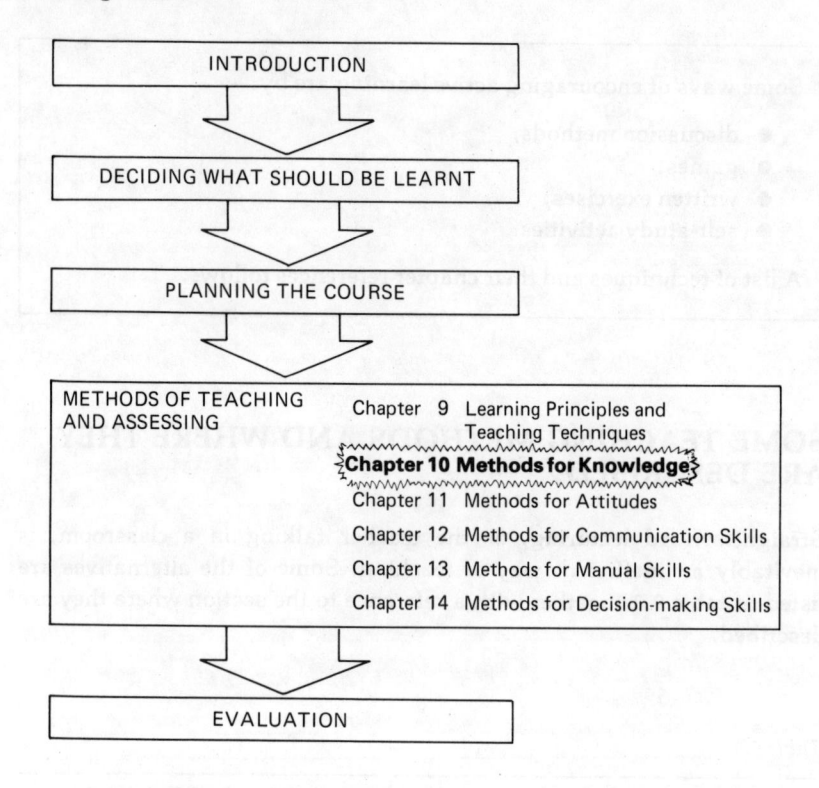

```
┌─────────────────────┐
│    INTRODUCTION     │
└──────────┬──────────┘
           ▼
┌─────────────────────────────┐
│ DECIDING WHAT SHOULD BE LEARNT │
└──────────┬──────────────────┘
           ▼
┌─────────────────────┐
│  PLANNING THE COURSE │
└──────────┬──────────┘
           ▼
┌────────────────────────┬──────────────────────────────────────────┐
│ METHODS OF TEACHING    │ Chapter  9  Learning Principles and      │
│ AND ASSESSING          │             Teaching Techniques          │
│                        │ **Chapter 10 Methods for Knowledge**     │
│                        │ Chapter 11  Methods for Attitudes        │
│                        │ Chapter 12  Methods for Communication Skills │
│                        │ Chapter 13  Methods for Manual Skills    │
│                        │ Chapter 14  Methods for Decision-making Skills │
└──────────┬─────────────┴──────────────────────────────────────────┘
           ▼
┌─────────────────────┐
│     EVALUATION      │
└─────────────────────┘
```

CONTENTS

10.1	What do we Mean by 'Knowledge'?	121
10.2	The Importance of Knowledge	122
10.3	The Functions of a Teacher in Helping Students Acquire Knowledge	123
10.4	Selecting Relevant and Necessary Knowledge	123
10.5	Establishing Sources of Information	126
10.6	Helping Students to Learn the Knowledge	128
10.7	Presenting Information Effectively	128
10.8	Helping Students to Remember Facts	132
10.9	Helping Students to Refer to Information Sources	133
10.10	Assessing Knowledge	134
10.11	Oral Examinations	135
10.12	Written Examinations	136
10.13	Open Book Examinations	140

10
Teaching and Assessing Knowledge

10.1 WHAT DO WE MEAN BY 'KNOWLEDGE'?

In this book, we use the word 'knowledge' to mean the facts, and the understanding of these facts, which will help the Primary Health Care (PHC) worker to give good health care to the community.

The range of knowledge which is relevant to health care is very wide—much wider than was thought even a few years ago. At one time the whole emphasis of health care was on treating the individual patient who was ill. This patient was thought of as a biological and chemical machine. So health workers were taught in great detail about the biology and chemistry of individual people (i.e. Anatomy, Physiology and Biochemistry). Since that time much more has been understood about the psychological and social causes of disease, so medicine is now much more concerned with the 'Whole Patient'. Also the policy of PHC has meant that educating patients, preventing disease and working with communities has become more important.

Because of these changes, the knowledge which is important to health workers has expanded to include knowledge about:

- communities and the way they work;
- psychology and methods of communication with individuals and groups;
- management and planning of health services;
- disease transmission and its control;
- providing suitable food and water.

This change in our understanding of health care does not mean that Anatomy and Physiology are of no value. But it does mean that these subjects are not the only foundation on which health care training should be built. It also means that learning large amounts of very detailed information on Anatomy and Physiology can be rather a waste of time.

Changing Facts

There are many 'facts' which are not really facts at all. They are just the present day opinion, or the best information we have so far. For example, the ways in which various diseases are treated change as new information becomes available.

Because facts change, teachers should make a special effort to continue their own education so that they are as well informed as possible. They should also emphasise to their students that 'facts' can change and that the students should continue learning throughout their career.

Naturally, there is little point in saying to students 'continue learning through your career', if the students are not taught how to learn by themselves. Therefore, there is a need to show students how to gain their own information from experience, books and colleagues. The students will not be able to do this if there is a heavy emphasis on lecturing during the training programme.

10.2 THE IMPORTANCE OF KNOWLEDGE

Obviously, knowledge is very important. If a health worker does not know the symptoms of a disease or the methods of constructing a well, then he cannot diagnose the disease or build a well.

However, knowledge is not enough.

Health workers must be able to apply the knowledge which they have and they must also have the manual skills and attitudes which are also absolutely essential in effective PHC. Therefore this book has separate chapters on these other important areas.

Many training programmes can be criticised as emphasising knowledge so much that the application of this knowledge, manual skills and attitudes are overlooked or are not given enough time in the curriculum. A proper balance is required in the curriculum between the time devoted to learning facts and the time spent in learning how to apply the facts.

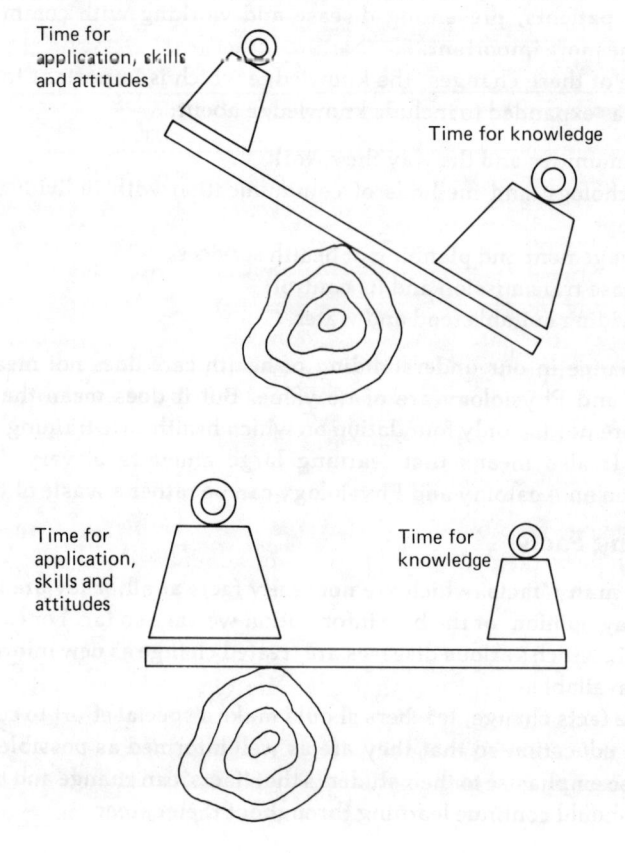

Figure 10.1 A better balance

Another criticism is that the old pattern was to teach the facts first and then teach students how to use them. This is an understandable error as there is logic in the argument 'you cannot teach students how to apply facts until they know the facts which they have to apply'.

But an alternative which is generally better is to learn the facts and how to apply them at the same time. This helps the learning of the facts themselves because they are seen to be useful and they are also rehearsed or revised at the time when they are applied.

10.3 THE FUNCTIONS OF A TEACHER IN HELPING STUDENTS ACQUIRE KNOWLEDGE

In helping students acquire knowledge a teacher needs to do more than simply go to a classroom and give a lesson.

He needs to:

- select relevant and necessary knowledge (section 10.4);
- establish sources of available information (section 10.5);
- help the student learn the facts in the best way possible;
- assess the level of knowledge acquired by the student.

In this chapter we discuss these functions.

10.4 SELECTING RELEVANT AND NECESSARY KNOWLEDGE

The selection of knowledge from the vast store available forms one of the most difficult decisions any teacher has to make. It is also one of the most important. The success of the health worker on the job will depend on his knowledge being relevant to the job. His success may also depend on him not being confused by learning an excess of unnecessary facts.

In selecting knowledge, a teacher needs to consider several factors—what the student already knows, his level of education and literacy, the length of training—but, above all, knowledge is selected *to enable the health worker to perform a task*. But even if we say 'Select the knowledge needed to perform a task the answer is not easy. Which knowledge is really necessary and how much?

It is possible to teach people simple skills without knowledge of what they are doing. But this is not desirable. For example, a nurse-aide or orderly might be taught to weigh babies or administer oral polio vaccine without any knowledge of nutrition or immunisation. This is certainly not recommended.

In general, people like to have knowledge. People like to understand the world they live in and to have reasons for the things which they do. Health workers work better and with more interest when they understand the reason for the task and how it will help the patient.

While there is general agreement that all health workers need some knowledge, there is very wide disagreement concerning the question 'how much knowledge needs to be remembered and understood by any particular category of worker;'.

The answer often given to this question by teachers in schools and colleges throughout the world is:

'as much as the average student can remember in the time available'!!

Teachers do not say this in those words, but this is the only interpretation which can explain what teachers do. This practice results mainly from a written competitive examination system, which depends on memory. Teachers pour knowledge into students' notebooks and students learn it and repeat it back in tests and examinations. The written examination system has resulted in an excess of remembered factual knowledge—at the expense of thinking, decision making, judgement, communication and practical skills.

One of the world's great educators, Paulo Freire, has called this the 'banking system of education'. Knowledge is gathered by the students in large amounts and stored away like money in a bank. Often it is left there, deep in the cellars of the mind and never used for the rest of his life!

What Process Can a Teacher Use to Select Relevant Knowledge?

The basic process teachers use to decide whether knowledge is relevant is Task Analysis. The way in which teachers can use this process is described in chapters 3, 4 and 6.

The general principle underlying the use of task analysis is:

> The amount of knowledge needed, is the amount necessary for a health worker to perform the task competently. This will include making rational decisions and judgements about the task

When this principle is applied, it is important to define the task precisely and to take into account who will be doing it. For example, 'dealing with anaemia in pregnancy' will be a different task to different levels of health worker. Thus the different levels of health worker will need different amounts of knowledge (see table 10.1).

It can be seen from table 10.1 that the more clearly a task is defined, the easier it becomes to determine the relevant knowledge.

Does this Procedure 'Restrict' a Health Worker's Knowledge?

A common argument against the task analysis approach is that it 'deprives' the learner of his basic right to wide, broad and deep knowledge! If this were true, it would be a reasonable objection.

No person should prevent others from learning. No teacher can be justified in confining students to minimum knowledge.

Table 10.1

Health worker	Task	Knowledge needed
MCH-aide in a village	Treat pregnant women for clinical anaemia	Signs and symptoms of anaemia in pregnancy Local foods containing iron Dosage of iron tablets
Community nurse in a Health Centre	Treat pregnant women for clinical anaemia Refer when necessary	As above, plus: Knowledge of several causes of anaemia Doses of iron and folic acid Treatment of hookworm and malaria Knowledge of levels of anaemia in relation to the stages of pregnancy
Medical assistant in charge of an area	Recognise the prevalence of anaemia in pregnancy in his area Advise on prevention	As above, plus: Knowledge of simple survey methods Knowledge of possible factors associated with high prevalence Knowledge of preventive measures available against main factors such as hookworm, malaria, malnutrition

While we agree that each person should know as much as possible about his work, we think that before he learns 'as much as possible', he should learn 'what is essential to do the job'.

Relevant knowledge defines what *every* student *must know* in order to do his job well. Relevant knowledge defines the core of essential knowledge.

After this core has been achieved teachers and students may expand knowledge as widely as their interests lead them.

This idea has been expressed as the Target Concept. This divides knowledge into 3 categories—must know, helpful to know, nice to know.

While it is true that 'knowing as much as possible' is generally a good thing, this only applies when the learner actively wishes to know.

Making students learn an excess of facts in order to pass examinations has many disadvantages.

- Learning facts does not help a worker to use them. For example, learning a description of a rare disease which he has not seen is unlikely to help in recognising the disease.
- Learning too many facts takes time away from learning practical skills.
- When inexperienced students are given facts to learn they cannot distinguish between what is essential and what is unimportant. By using the target concept a teacher can guide students into essential learning.
- Learning unnecessary facts penalises the less bright students. These students may be able to perform well by learning the core of relevant

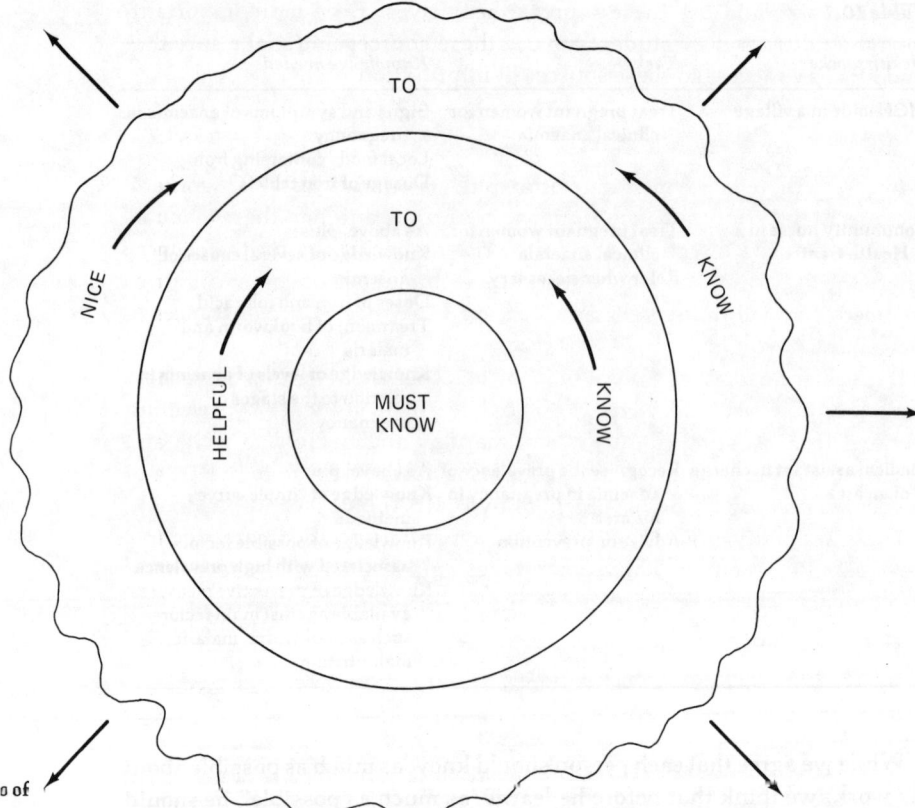

Figure 10.2 Disadvantages of learning unnecessary facts

knowledge—leaving the brighter students to pick up the 'nice to know' knowledge.
- It has been found by experience that a large percentage of facts learned doing a training course are forgotten and unused by experienced and competent workers in the field. This suggests that learning unnecessary facts is a waste of time and effort. How much of your initial training in anatomy can you remember now?

10.5 ESTABLISHING SOURCES OF INFORMATION

As mentioned in section 10.1, health knowledge is continuously expanding. Approaches to Primary Health Care and how it is best applied are changing rapidly as world-wide experience in this field accumulates. A teacher cannot rely on the knowledge which he gained during his own studies—or even on the experience he has gained since. So he must keep his own knowledge up-to-date.

The main sources for information which will allow the teacher to keep up-to-date are:

- Manuals.
- Books, journals and newsletters (library).
- Other people.

Teachers should use these sources themselves. Even more important, they should train their students to use these sources and make sure that students have access to these sources of information.

Manuals

Nowadays there is a wide range of manuals available for PHC workers. Because PHC differs so much from one country to another, these manuals can only be used directly if they are written specifically for the country where the PHC workers will be working. If manuals from other countries are used they will need to be adapted to fit the special circumstances of each country.

It is easier to adapt a manual than write a new one. A group of teachers could get together and write a manual for their students by selecting sections from existing manuals and adapting them. How to write and duplicate teaching materials and manuals is described simply in Part 4 of the book *Teaching for Better Learning* by F. R. Abbatt (see Appendix 1).

There are many advantages in having a manual specifically related to a particular PHC course. These advantages apply both for the teacher and the students. These are:

- The teacher knows exactly what to teach.
- The student knows exactly what to learn.
- It releases the student from the burden of taking detailed notes in lectures.
- It saves the teacher the burden of making too many handouts.
- It makes it easier for a new teacher to take over from another teacher who has left or is ill.
- It develops standards of knowledge and procedures in PHC for the country.
- It assists fair assessment by examiners.
- A local manual is cheap to produce and can be revised frequently to keep up with changing circumstances.

Books, Journals and Newsletters

It is the responsibility of Principals of schools, together with their teachers, to establish a library for use of both students and teachers.

A library should not only contain books, but also journals, pamphlets and local information and documents, such as annual reports of the Ministry of Health. A list of books relevant to PHC is to be found in Appendix 1. It should be noted that some journals and newsletters are free.

Certain international agencies may grant funds to help establish a library, for example, UNICEF or The British Council.

Other People

In most areas of the world there are people with knowledge and experience. Unfortunately, most people don't talk about their experiences unless specifically asked to do so.

For example, a PHC teacher in a new area may wish to know more about the community. This will be gained over time. But there may be a knowledgeable priest or schoolteacher who can give more information in one evening's conversation than can be gained in a year of observation. This will be particularly true if the local language is unknown to the new teacher. Workers in other government departments may also be information sources—agricultural workers may know about types of food grown, sisters in rural clinics may know about local health beliefs.

When a PHC teacher finds a person who can contribute in this way he can invite them to share their knowledge with his students.

A great deal of the knowledge needed in PHC is about people, their customs and way of life—this knowledge cannot be found in books.

Another source of information is the 'Subject Matter Expert'. These are people who know a great deal about one field, for example, a university lecturer or a consultant in a hospital. Such people often have difficulty in teaching students with less education because they are unable to talk in a simple, straightforward manner. But they are very good at giving information which is correct and up-to-date. The PHC teacher can then put this information in a form understood by his students.

10.6 HELPING STUDENTS TO LEARN THE KNOWLEDGE

A teacher selects the knowledge needed to perform a task well, by doing a task analysis. This knowledge will be taught within the classroom situation and during practical work in relation to the relevant tasks. The selected knowledge must be presented to the student.

Health workers need to remember a great number of facts to work effectively. But there are also facts which they need to use but need not remember—provided they can be taught to 'look things up' in information sources. For example, it is better to have a drug dosage book than to expect students to learn the doses of all the main drugs. It is also safer for the patient.

Teachers need to:

- present information effectively (section 10.7);
- help students remember facts (section 10.8);
- help students refer to information sources (section 10.9).

10.7 PRESENTING INFORMATION EFFECTIVELY

The principles of effective presentation have been described in chapter 9. It will be remembered that this can be summarised as:

Clarity,
Relevance to the future,
Relevance to previous experience, and
Structure.

Also a good presentation needs to be supported by the active participation of, and feedback to, the students.

Some techniques to achieve effective presentation are described below.

(i) Using Visual Aids

Traditional teaching is based on a belief that when we speak, others hear, understand and remember all we say. This is not so. Some educators claim that we remember only 10–20% of what we hear.

Students are well aware that they will not remember much. That is why they insist on taking notes in class.

Talking is one of the least effective ways of presenting information. A great deal more is learned and remembered when the information is given in the form of pictures, slide shows, films or models, that is, by using visual aids.

The blackboard, the overhead projector or the flip chart are tools for presenting visual materials in the classroom—whether as the written word or diagrams. The skilful use of these tools is important for effective presentation of information.

(ii) Using the Chalkboard

The chalkboard (blackboard) is the most universal visual aid. It is frequently used badly and ineffectively.

Certain rules should be observed by teachers using the chalkboard and these are listed here.

- Never talk and write on the blackboard at the same time. When a teacher talks whilst facing the blackboard his words cannot be heard. Also since speech is faster than writing, what he is saying will be ahead of what he is writing. The student then has to think of two things at once—what is being written and what is being said. Very few people can manage this.
- Writing on the board should be legible and visible at the back of the class.
- What is placed on the board should be selective. For example, a new word, which needs to be spelt; a single point which is being emphasised; a diagram around which the lesson revolves; a summary of what has been said; a compiling of major points which will become a summary at the end of the lesson.
- What is on the board should relate to what is being explained at that time. When the topic changes previous items should be wiped off the board. This very important point is often ignored. Sometimes one finds teachers searching for small spaces on a crowded blackboard to write up some new information—the whole board being a scrawling confusion.
- Visual items draw attention to themselves. If the item does not coincide with what is being said, it will detract from attention to the spoken word. On the other hand, if the item on the board illustrates

what is being said, then it will reinforce the spoken word and focus attention.
- Diagrams on the board should be as simple as possible. Detailed, complex diagrams add to confusion, instead of clarifying.
- If a good diagram is very important to the lesson, it should be drawn carefully beforehand, or drawn by a student who can draw well. This is to save time during the class period. Alternatively a diagram could be drawn on a large card and pinned to the frame of the blackboard.

(iii) Using the Overhead Projector

There are many advantages to the overhead projector but the main one is that the teacher can face the class and talk at the same time as he writes or draws.

The same rules listed above for the chalkboard apply equally to the overhead projector. Items, whether words or diagrams, should be selective, clear, visible, simple and coincide with what the speaker is saying.

A further advantage of the overhead projector is that permanent transparencies can be prepared and preserved in cardboard frames for future use.

(iv) Using a Slide Projector

Transparent slides projected on a screen can be used in two ways. Either in teaching groups of students or whole classes, or for individuals to study with the help of a guide-sheet.

In the classroom, slides should be presented with clearly stated objectives. It is easy to substitute a slide-show for teaching—that is to spend a class period showing slides one after another and talking about them, without a clearly formulated learning objective for the lesson.

All visual aids are adjuncts to an educational purpose, and need to be selected with care and used as a learning experience, or to reinforce a learning experience.

One of the best uses of transparent slides is for individual study. A programme can be prepared in which the student is asked questions concerning each slide to which he writes down the answers. Later he corrects his own answers from an answer sheet. If he has made a mistake he can return and study the slide again. In this way he can practise active recall and gain immediate feedback.

(Teachers needing more information on Visual Communication are referred to the book *Visual Communication* by Denys Saunders, given in Appendix 1. The use of visuals is a large subject and outside the scope of this book.)

(v) Learning Facts by Self-study

Students very rarely learn all the facts they need during the class session where the information is presented. They are too busy trying to understand the new material—or else too busy taking notes! Normally, students learn facts during their private study periods—they learn from manuals or handouts or their own notes.

Because students do not learn many facts during class sessions it is not a good use of time to spend these periods passing facts from the blackboard to the students' notebooks. It is better to spend class time in discussing the difficult points of a topic and to give students the facts to learn during their study periods. Facts can be given to students either by asking them to read a section of a manual (if a suitable one is available) or by giving them handouts.

A difficult situation arises when no duplicator for making handouts is available, or where there is insufficient paper. A teacher can write short notes making several carbon copies. These can be given to groups of students to copy into their notebooks—during their self-study periods, not during class time.

> It is a waste of valuable teaching time to spend it in copying notes

There are a number of techniques which encourage students to study without a teacher—sometimes known as 'Self-instructional Programmes'.

All these methods require a great deal of preparation time on the part of the teacher. But after the original preparation, the student studies on his own and the teacher's role is to help him over difficulties and assess his progress. These methods can only be used with literate students sufficiently advanced to learn through reading.

In a self-instructional programme, the student is given something to do. It might be to read a certain section, or to look at a slide or to perform a task. After this, he is asked questions concerning the matter which he corrects himself by using an answer sheet. When he has completed one topic or 'unit' he is assessed by the teacher. If he passes this assessment, he then proceeds to the next topic. In this way, proceeding step by step, he masters the whole subject.

Self-instruction need not involve a whole programme. A teacher could prepare a self-instruction unit for just one lesson or one practical.

One of the main advantages of self-instruction is that it gives the student confidence in his ability to learn by himself. It 'weans' him from dependence on the teacher.

(vi) Handouts

Handouts are duplicated papers given out by teachers to students either to:

- act as guides for work to be done or references to be looked up; or
- to remind students of the main points of a lesson or learning experience.

Handouts should not be used as substitutes for manuals, texts and references.

A handout is both a visual material which aids learning and an adjunct to self-study.

Since students learn from handouts, revise from handouts and refer to them frequently it is important that they are prepared with care, and have a clear purpose.

Statements and spelling should be accurate.
Statements should be consistent with the other texts or manuals students are using.
If a topic is controversial, this should be stated.
Each handout should have a clear objective/purpose.
If a handout is giving instructions for practical work, these should be complete and specific.

All the criteria which apply to presentation of information in class also apply to handouts, that is:

clarity;
relevance to the future;
relevance to previous experience; and
structure.

There are two aspects of 'structure' which are significant in a handout. First the ideas should be arranged in a logical order or sequence. The order of arrangement will be the way it is remembered by the student—if the presentation is confused, his memory will be confused. The other aspect of structure is the layout. This is the arrangement of words, headings and diagrams on the page. The layout helps learning if it is clear, and if important points 'stand out'—by being put in capitals, or surrounded by a box—or underlined or given space.

10.8 HELPING STUDENTS TO REMEMBER FACTS

(i) Using Recall

Some teachers believe that students learn when statements are repeated over and over again. This is more likely to produce boredom than learning.

> Recall by the student is more effective for remembering than repetition by the teacher

In a jungle or a field of grass, the more often somebody walks through it, the easier it becomes to pass along. Similarly, the more often a student recalls information, the easier it becomes to do so.

Active recall of information 'makes a pathway in the mind'.
How can teachers encourage students to 'recall'?

- Ask questions frequently during each session.
- Ask questions each day about yesterday's lessons.
- Ask questions each week about last week's lessons.

- Encourage students to work in pairs and ask each other questions.
- Giving frequent short tests and correcting the answers immediately in class. Get the students to correct their own or each other's questions.
- Recalling the information when doing the practical task to which the 'knowledge' is related.

(ii) Using the Information

As explained in chapter 9, one of the best ways of learning is active learning.

The ideal situation is to do the actual task to which the learning relates as soon as possible after the information is presented. This is often not practical.

But it is possible for students to use the information by doing exercises which require them to apply the knowledge learned.

Case studies and patient management problems are common simulations through which students can learn to apply knowledge. These are discussed in more detail in the chapter on Decision-making Skills (chapter 14).

10.9 HELPING STUDENTS TO REFER TO INFORMATION SOURCES

It has been mentioned in section 6.2 that health information changes rapidly and that health workers need to learn continually throughout life.

An important job of the teacher is to train students how to find information for themselves.

This can be done by using methods of graded difficulty:

- Ask a question and let the student look it up in a given reference.
- Ask several questions to be looked up in several references.
- Ask questions. Let the students search for the reference in the index of books.
- Give the students 'blank' notes with only the headings written out. Let the students make their own notes by referring to information sources.
- Give students a 'project' to do which would require them to find out information from several sources.

PHC workers need encouragement to use handbooks, manuals and other reference sources. Many have become used to the school system where information is provided only through the teacher. But with encouragement and training, even primary school leavers will enjoy searching out information for themselves.

Flowcharts for diagnosis, management schedules, drug dosage tables and procedure techniques are major reference materials which need to be available for use in clinics and health centres. For cultural reasons, PHC workers often refuse to use reference sources in the clinic situation. Not to know 'everything' is regarded as 'shameful' in front of patients. But a chart on the wall, or a book on the shelf beside the worker can be referred to without the patient's knowledge. If students are encouraged to 'look things up' during training, and especially if the teacher himself uses references, students will soon become used to the idea. It will become a habit to be used throughout life.

10.10 ASSESSING KNOWLEDGE

The principles of assessment described in chapter 8 can usefully be applied to the assessment of knowledge. In particular the idea of validity concerns the relationship between the assessment and the field situation in which the knowledge is used. So examinations which require students to remember minute details of dosages of drugs which are rarely used are not valid. This is because in the field, the PHC worker should look up these dosages. Therefore a better examination would test whether the health worker could use the reference books or manuals available in the field, rather than testing memory.

Reliability will be high when a student's mark reflects his real ability. This will be unlikely to happen when students are asked to write essays, because these only sample a small part of the student's knowledge and because different examiners often mark to very different standards. A better way is to use short-answer questions or multiple-choice questions, which can be marked more objectively and which sample a greater range of knowledge.

What Knowledge Should be Assessed?

The knowledge to be assessed should be the knowledge which is essential to perform health care tasks. One should not bother to assess the tiny details or the trivia. The essential knowledge is the 'core' or 'target' knowledge which has been derived through the process of task analysis. It is the same knowledge which has been the focus of the teaching.

Because the knowledge to be tested is the essential knowledge, it follows that the pass marks should be high. Fifty per cent is clearly far too low a pass mark if the assessment is only dealing with important facts. Possibly 80% or even 90% would be a more appropriate pass standard.

When Should Knowledge be Assessed?

Assessing the students' mastery of the knowledge helps learning. So the assessment should take place frequently as a way of helping learning. This is enhanced when combined with immediate feedback—either by rapid verbal affirmation or correction—or the rapid return of marked written answers.

Weekly, fortnightly or monthly written tests throughout a course are valuable both as learning aids and as monitors of progress for teachers and students.

One problem is that marking papers takes a great deal of teachers' time. This problem can be overcome if short-answer or multiple-choice questions are used. The papers can be marked immediately at the conclusion of the test—each student marking either his own, or his neighbour's paper. The correct answers are read out, by the teacher, in front of the class. Any queries from students or misunderstandings of the questions or the answer can be dealt with on the spot by the teacher. The students mark the papers according to the scoring system arranged by the teacher. This system can only be used when tests are used for learning. It is not fair to use student-marked papers in 'pass or fail' assessment.

In addition there should naturally be end-of-course assessments which should be marked by the teacher, or possibly by external examiners.

How Should the Assessment be Done?

One can assess whether a student 'has knowledge' in two main ways:

(1) Whether he can express knowledge in words—through oral (section 10.11) or written examinations (section 10.12).
(2) Whether he can apply and use knowledge—through practical examinations (see chapters 12–14).

In addition one can assess whether a student can 'refer to information sources':

(3) By the Open Book Examination (section 10.13).

10.11 ORAL EXAMINATIONS

This method has low reliability and low validity.

The reliability is low because the time restrictions mean that only a small percentage of a candidate's knowledge can be assessed. It is also unreliable because the questions may be worded in a way not understood by the candidate, there is wide variation in students' ability to express themselves verbally, the situation produces nervousness and anxiety, examiners may be biased by personal appearance and mannerisms, there is no clear, unequivocal scoring method and so on.

Validity is also low. This is because what the students are asked to do is so different from the work they will do in the field.

In the case of illiterate or semi-literate PHC workers who cannot write fluently, there is some grounds for using oral examinations in place of written methods. However, in this situation the major assessment should be based on observation of students doing practical work.

A way of conducting an oral examination which improves reliability is shown below. Reliability is improved because it ensures sampling questions from the whole course. Reliability is also improved by having carefully worded non-ambiguous questions, by using two examiners, by ensuring the student understands the questions, and using a rating scale attached to a specific scoring system.

The Improved Oral Examination

(1) Make a large series of cards. On each card write one factual question, carefully worded. (Check the wording by reading the questions to people who should know the answer—and seeing whether their answer implies that they have understood the question.)

(2) Divide the cards into groups, each group representing one section of the course.

(3) Use two examiners to assess each candidate.

(4) One or more cards are picked at random from each group, which ensures asking one or more questions from each part of the course.

(5) The examiner reads the question and repeats it if the candidate doesn't understand it. If the candidate is literate, the candidate himself reads the question aloud.

(6) After the candidate has answered the question, the examiner places a tick in an appropriate box on a pre-prepared rating scale.

(7) There is a scoring system related to the boxes, but this is unknown to the examiner.

Question No.	Answer complete and correct	Answer partial but correct	Answer partly right/ partly wrong	Answer confused	Does not know	Guesses wrong answer
1	✓					
2				✓		
3		✓				
4	✓					
etc.					✓	

10.12 WRITTEN EXAMINATIONS

There are three main varieties of written tests:

- multiple-choice questions (MCQs);
- essays;
- short-answer questions.

(i) Multiple-choice Questions (MCQs)

Multiple-choice questions come in many different forms. The most common are the 'One-from five' type and the 'multiple true–false' type. The 'one-from-five' type consists of a single statement (known as the stem) followed by a number of choices (usually five). Only one of the five choices is correct. Incorrect choices are known as *distractors*—they should be reasonably plausible to a person who lacks the knowledge to be tested. But they should be clearly wrong to a student who has the knowledge.

In the 'multiple true–false' type the stem is followed by a series of statements, each of which may be true or may be false. The student indicates whether in his opinion the statement is true or not.

Examples of multiple-choice questions are shown below. These examples have been adapted from the book *Primary Child Care*, Vol. 2, by

Maurice King. There are 1000 multiple-choice questions concerning child care in this book and a PHC teacher who is training child care health workers could use some of them.

Examples of 'One from Five' Type Multiple-choice Questions

(1) Bianca has a severe hookworm infection. In which of these ways was she probably infected?
    A. Faeces to mouth
    B. By larvae going through her skin
    C. By inhaling infected droplets
    D. By contact
    E. By a dirty needle

(2) Rosario (3 yrs, 18 kg, 37.4°C) for the last few weeks has had several liquid stools each day. They are frothy with bubbles of gas and have an abnormal smell. There is no blood in his stools. He is mildly ill and is not dehydrated. Unfortunately your clinic has no microscope to examine his stools. What is his most probable diagnosis?
    A. Bacillary dysentery
    B. Amoebic dysentery
    C. Giardiasis
    D. The chronic diarrhoea of malnutrition

Examples of True–False Type Multiple-choice Questions

(1) Bianca has a severe hookworm infection. The way in which she was infected could have been

A.	Faeces to mouth	True	False
B.	By larvae through the skin	True	False
C.	By inhaling infected droplets	True	False
D.	By contact	True	False
E.	By a dirty needle	True	False

(2) Rosario (3 yrs, 18 kg, 37.4°C) for the last few weeks has had several liquid stools each day. They are frothy with bubbles of gas and have an abnormal smell. There is no blood in his stools. He is mildly ill and is not dehydrated. Unfortunately, your clinic has no microscope to examine his stools. What is his most probable diagnosis?

A.	Bacillary dysentery	True	False
B.	Amoebic dysentery	True	False
C.	Giardiasis	True	False
D.	The chronic diarrhoea of malnutrition	True	False

Notice that in the one-from-five type one answer must be selected. So if a student knows one answer is correct, the rest can be ignored. On the other hand, in the true–false type, even if the student knows one statement is true, he must look at each of the other statements and make up his mind in every case.

Notice also that although the first type is called 'one-from-five', it is possible to only have three distractors or even to have five distractors. In the true–false type any number of statements can follow each stem (though it is common to always have five).

The most suitable marking scheme for the one-from-five type is to give one mark for each correct answer. Wrong answers can either be given 0 or sometimes $-1/4$. Marking the true–false type is best done by giving 1 for a right answer (whether the right answer is 'true' or 'false') and -1 for a wrong answer. (In a paper with a lot of statements this marking scheme compensates for guessing.)

On balance, if MCQs are used, it is better to use the true–false type as these test more knowledge in a given time, are no more affected by guessing than the other type (though a lot of people do not realise this), and are easier to write because the teacher does not have to think of as many plausible distractors.

MCQs are reliable. There is little doubt about the correct answer. Whoever marks the paper the score will be identical. Marking is quick and simple. It can be done by a clerk or a layman who doesn't know the subject.

MCQs also increase reliability because they can assess a large part of the course material in a short time. But sometimes validity is decreased—if the questions concentrate on rare or trivial points.

Unfortunately, even though the ideal MCQ test has high reliability it has several serious disadvantages. These tests are very difficult to set. So the quick marking time is offset by the long composing time. Very often the distractors are so obviously wrong, that the correct answer is obvious. In this case there is really no choice, and furthermore the correct answer is already there presented to the candidate. He does not even have to remember it!

Unless PHC teachers are very experienced at making MCQs or unless they are taken from an authoritative book, we do not recommend their use in assessing health workers.

(ii) Essays

These are a traditional form of assessment. It has been customary for an examination to consist of four or five questions to be answered in 2 hours or so at the end of one year's work. This method has low validity because it assesses only the ability to repeat knowledge—not the ability to use it. It also has very low reliability, because the questions are not very specific and different examiners score answers widely differently, because the mark may depend on quality of writing rather than the knowledge, and because the essays usually only cover a small proportion of the course.

This method is not suitable for PHC assessment. Very few PHC workers can write fast or express themselves clearly through the written word. These deficiencies add to its unreliability.

The authors believe that the essay-type examination should not be used for assessing PHC workers.

(iii) Short-answer Questions

This method requires answers to be expressed as either:

single words, or
one or more simple sentences.

The question specifically states the number of points required in the answer and the question is scored on the number of points answered correctly.

A large number of questions can be answered in a short time which increases course coverage. This will increase reliability. The method is also reliable because the scoring is based on a clearly defined number of points. But because the answers are in sentences composed by the candidates, there will be a variability in the precision of answers—even though they may be substantially correct. This makes short-answer questions rather less reliable than MCQs—but on the other hand, they are much easier to compose.

Some examples of short-answer questions are shown below.

This seems an appropriate method to use with literate PHC workers.

If short-answer questions are used with actual examples of clinical case histories, they can become patient management problems. This enormously increases validity because a patient management problem deals with actual situations.

Examples of Short-answer Questions

(1) Mention three causes of blood-stained faeces in a child
   a. ─────────────────────────
   b. ─────────────────────────
   c. ─────────────────────────   3 marks

(2) A drug called Piperazine is used for 2 different intestinal worms.
   A. Name the two worms
   a. ─────────────────────────
   b. ─────────────────────────   2 marks
   B. What is the daily dose of piperazine
   a. in a child aged 8 years ───────────
   b. in an adult ──────────────────   2 marks
   C. How many days would you give treatment for
   a. worm you named under (a) above ──────
   b. worm you named under (b) above ────── 2 marks

> (3) Karim aged 4 years has had sore, red, watery eyes for several days. There is no pus in the eyes. He has no fever and is otherwise well. Several other villagers have the same symptoms.
>
>   a. Give a possible diagnosis ——————
>   b. Explain your treatment ——————
>   ——————————————————
>   —————————————— 5 marks

Patient-management problems are described in detail in the chapter on Decision-making Skills (chapter 14).

10.13 OPEN BOOK EXAMINATIONS

In this type of assessment, all the books and other information the student will need to answer the questions are made available to him in the examination hall. He has to answer a set of questions during a fixed time period.

If this method is used to assess a student's ability to find information from reference sources, it will only be valid if he does *not* know the answers to the questions asked.

The reliability will depend on the type of test, that is on whether it is an objective type of test (multiple-choice or short-answer) or an essay.

Sometimes this method is used in testing problem-solving ability. In this case, it will be assessing two separate skills—the ability to solve problems (to decide which questions to look up) and the ability to use reference material.

SUMMARY

- Students should remember facts, but it is also important for them to be able to look up information and apply the information which they have learnt.
- Teachers can help learning by:
    selecting the most important and relevant facts;
    establishing sources of information;
    presenting the information effectively.
- Effective presentation is:
    clear;
    made relevant to future work and past experience;
    well structured.
- Presentations can be made more visual by using:
    the chalkboard, overhead projector, slides and films.
- The knowledge to be assessed should be that core of essential knowledge which has been selected through task analysis.
- All students should be shown to have mastered most of this knowledge (the pass-mark should be high).
- Knowledge is assessed by oral and written tests *and* during practical examinations.
- The main methods which can be used to assess knowledge in the classroom setting are:
    Oral examinations.
    One-from-five and true–false multiple-choice questions.
    Essays.
    Short-answer questions.
    Patient management problems.
- Oral examinations should only be used for illiterate candidates and then in combination with practical examinations.
- Essays have low reliability and low validity and should not be used.
- Multiple-choice type questions have high reliability but are very difficult to compose successfully. They are not recommended.
- Short-answer questions seem suitable for assessing PHC workers.
- Open book examinations assess whether students can use references.
- Assessment helps learning particularly when combined with immediate feedback.

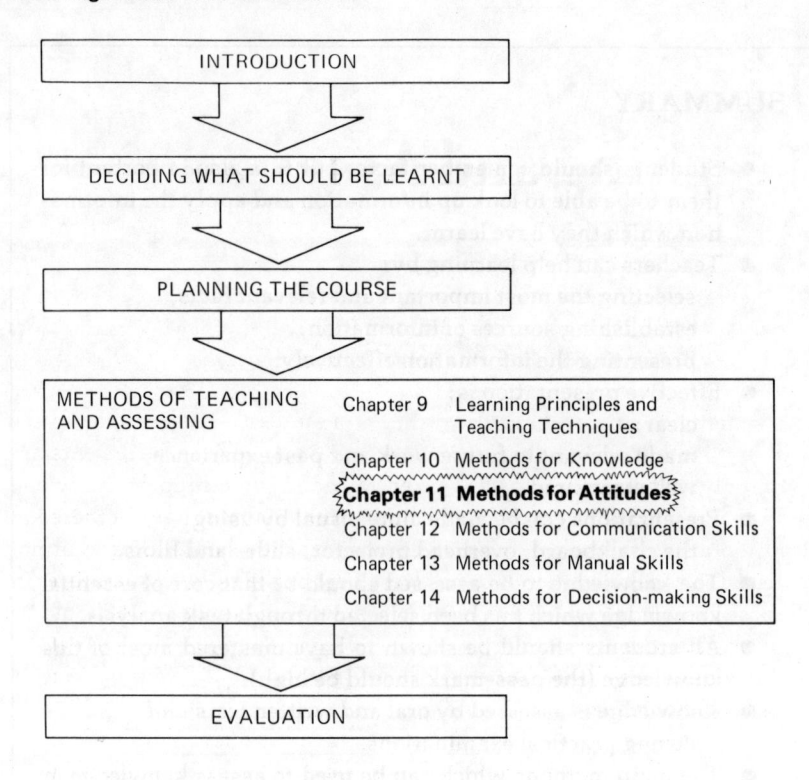

```
        ┌─────────────────────┐
        │   INTRODUCTION      │
        └─────────┬───────────┘
                  ▼
        ┌─────────────────────────────┐
        │ DECIDING WHAT SHOULD BE LEARNT │
        └─────────┬───────────────────┘
                  ▼
        ┌─────────────────────┐
        │  PLANNING THE COURSE │
        └─────────┬───────────┘
                  ▼
```

METHODS OF TEACHING AND ASSESSING	Chapter 9	Learning Principles and Teaching Techniques
	Chapter 10	Methods for Knowledge
	Chapter 11	**Methods for Attitudes**
	Chapter 12	Methods for Communication Skills
	Chapter 13	Methods for Manual Skills
	Chapter 14	Methods for Decision-making Skills

```
                  ▼
        ┌─────────────────────┐
        │     EVALUATION      │
        └─────────────────────┘
```

CONTENTS

11.1	What are Attitudes?	143
11.2	Are Attitudes Important?	144
11.3	Can Attitudes be Taught?	145
11.4	What Attitudes should be Taught?	146
11.5	Methods of Teaching Attitudes	146
11.6	Telling Students about Attitudes	147
11.7	Encouraging Students to Discuss Attitudes	148
11.8	Providing Information and Experience	149
11.9	Providing Role Models and Examples	150
11.10	Using Role-play Exercises	151
11.11	Some Examples of Role Plays	154
11.12	Assessing Attitudes	154

11
Teaching and Assessing Attitudes

11.1 WHAT ARE ATTITUDES?

It is sometimes said of a health worker or a student, 'His attitude is very bad' or, 'He has a very good attitude to his work'. These statements are commonly made after a health worker has done something specially bad or specially good. For example a health worker may not have bothered to keep the dispensary clean, or arrived very late at a health centre, or not bothered to check whether vaccines were kept at the right temperature. In all these cases it is assumed that the health worker *knows* what should be done, and has the necessary *skill* to do it. What has gone wrong is that the health worker has not used his knowledge and skill. This is seen as evidence of an unsatisfactory attitude.

These examples show the link between attitudes and performance or behaviour. In fact attitudes are perhaps best thought of as the driving forces which determine how people tend to behave or perform.

> Attitudes determine how a person tends to behave

This fairly simple idea is of course rather more complicated in real life. In a particular situation a person's actions are the result of several attitudes, and these attitudes may be conflicting. As an example, a health worker may be just setting off to run an immunisation clinic in a nearby village when a mother arrives with a sick child. The health worker may have attitudes which make it more likely that he will examine the child carefully and delay the clinic. These attitudes might be:

- concern for the mother and child;
- reluctance to travel;
- valuing of curative care.

On the other hand the health worker may have other attitudes which might make him hurry the examination or tell the mother to come back later. These attitudes might be:

- valuing promptness and a desire not to make the people wanting immunisations wait;
- valuing preventive care.

What the health worker actually does will be the result of the balance of these different attitudes.

Attitudes are rather different from knowledge and the three types of skills in several ways. First of all, they are rather vague and difficult to specify. (To illustrate this for yourself, you might try to write down 10 facts which health workers should know or 10 skills they should have. This will be fairly easy. Now try to write down 10 attitudes! This will be much more difficult.)

> Attitudes are difficult to define precisely

As a result of this difficulty, it is hard for teachers to know exactly what should be taught.

Another difference is that it is very difficult to find out what attitudes a person has. You can fairly easily find out whether a student knows the correct storage conditions for measles vaccine or has the skill to detect an enlarged spleen. It is much harder to find out whether a student has an attitude of respect for a patient's beliefs. This is because the attitude can only be deduced from the way a person behaves—and this behaviour is the result of several different attitudes.

> It is difficult to find out what a person's attitudes are

Finally, attitudes are not completely stable. They may change over a period of time—although there must be some degree of stability.

11.2 ARE ATTITUDES IMPORTANT?

Most health workers of all types and their teachers would probably agree that:

> Attitudes are very important

However, in Primary Health Care (PHC) the attitudes of the health worker are even more important than for hospital workers or those involved in curative clinical medicine.

Why is this?

At the specific and practical level, PHC workers often work in greater isolation, with less supervision and fewer rewards of prestige and money than other health workers. Therefore the temptation not to follow aseptic techniques rigorously or not to maintain standards is much greater.

A much more general point is that PHC is based on a philosophy and values which are quite different from the traditional Western Medicine. These differences are discussed in chapter 1, but two examples will illustrate this point. PHC should develop a community's or an individual's ability to look after themselves. This ability depends on health workers sharing their knowledge and skills. To do this, the health workers must have communication skills—but they must also have the attitude which makes them want to communicate their knowledge and skills.

A second example is that PHC depends on providing a service for all members of the population. This means that health workers must be willing to live—and continue to live—in rural areas and the poorer areas

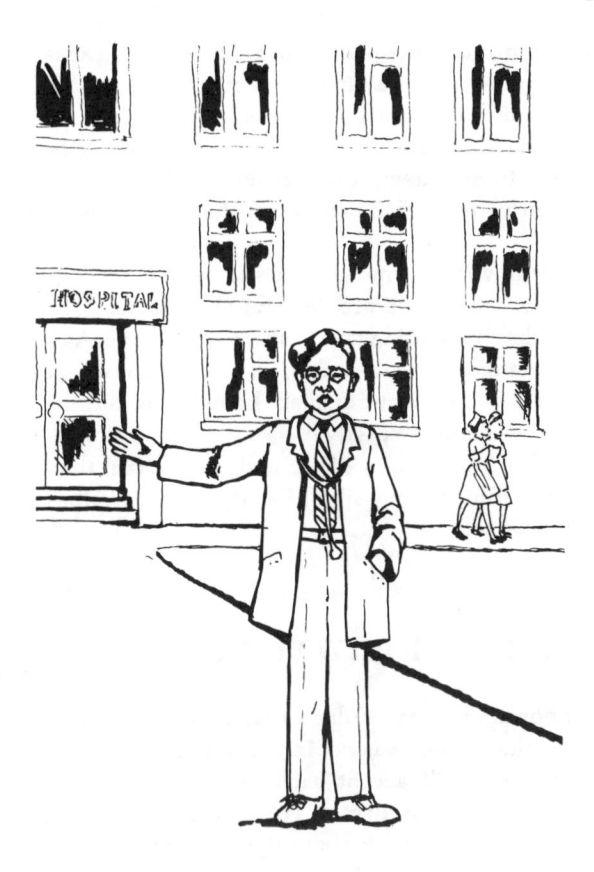

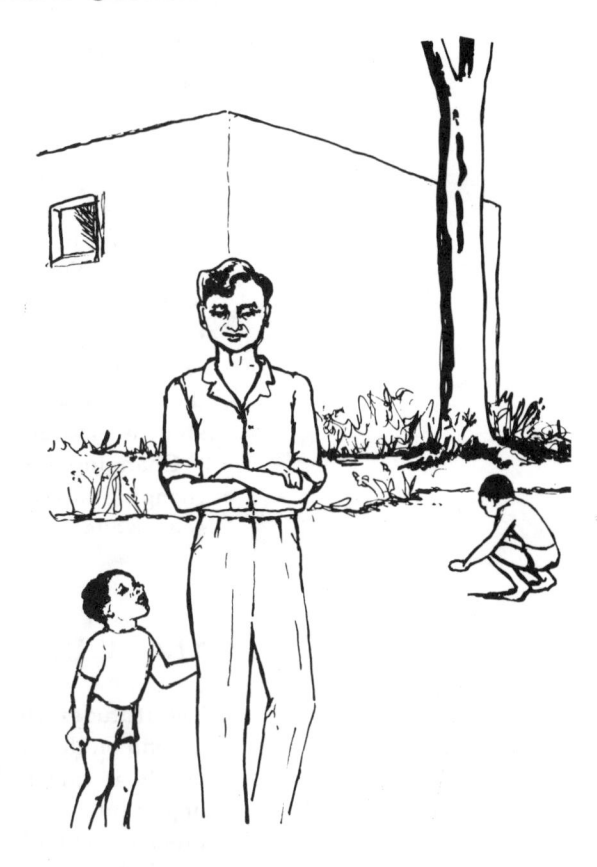

Figure 11.1 Doctors in hospitals have better technical facilities

Figure 11.2 Health workers in villages must have attitudes of service to the local community

of large cities. In the past it has always been difficult to find enough health workers with the attitudes which will lead to them continuing to work in the disadvantaged parts of a country.

> It is essential that PHC workers have attitudes which are consistent with the philosophy of PHC

11.3 CAN ATTITUDES BE TAUGHT?

Some people believe that attitudes are established at a very early age and that once the attitudes are established they cannot be changed. There does seem to be some truth in this idea. Certainly young children change attitudes much more readily than middle-aged adults. And it is also true that attitudes learnt in early childhood do tend to continue into adult life.

However, teachers who work with groups of students over a period of months or years will always be able to see changes in the students' attitudes taking place. Teachers will also be able to remember how their own attitudes have changed over the years.

Therefore changes in attitudes do take place—but can teachers cause this change of attitude? How much change can be expected?

Changes in attitude are quite different to changes in knowledge. A student who does not know how to make Oral Rehydration Fluid can be told the ingredients and how to mix them. The teacher can then test the student's knowledge and can be reasonably confident that the student's knowledge has changed.

On the other hand, a student who does not want to share his knowledge with the community is quite a different problem for the teacher. The teacher may tell the student that he should want to share knowledge. As a result the student may have changed his knowledge, i.e. he may know that the teacher says PHC workers should want to share knowledge. But the student's attitude is unlikely to change so easily.

Changing attitudes is much slower, less direct and less certain than changing knowledge or skills. But it is possible. Section 11.5 describes some ways in which it can be done.

11.4 WHAT ATTITUDES SHOULD BE TAUGHT?

The attitudes which are important in a particular situation will, of course, depend on that situation. So the list below is not intended to be complete, nor is it intended that teachers will accept each of the attitudes as important and appropriate for their students. The sole purpose is to provide a stimulus to help teachers to think about the kinds of attitudes which they would like their students to have by the end of the course.

Some attitudes appropriate in PHC include:

- A desire to continue learning throughout life.
- Respect for the convenience, comfort and beliefs of all patients.
- A desire to share knowledge and skills.
- An eagerness to overcome difficulties.
- A willingness to share in the whole range of community activities.
- A desire to be of service to the community and to individuals within the community.
- A desire to co-operate with other workers in the community.

11.5 METHODS OF TEACHING ATTITUDES

Teaching an attitude is quite different from teaching facts. You might start a teaching session on facts by saying, 'At the end of this session I expect that you will be able to describe the way in which trachoma is transmitted—and how it can be prevented'. On the other hand, it would not make sense to begin a teaching session by saying 'At the end of this session, you will be eager to share your knowledge and skills with the community'. Attitude change is usually slower than this. It is also usually the result of a whole series of experiences.

The teacher's job therefore is to provide a whole series of experiences for the student, which together will probably encourage the desired attitude change.

However, one difficulty is that experiences which students have may lead to unplanned attitude changes. For example, the need for promptness may be talked about by teachers. But if teachers often arrive late at sessions or if they take no action when students are persistently late, then the teacher's behaviour gives a conflicting message that promptness does not matter. A similar situation can arise when PHC workers are trained in cities and in large hospitals. They may be told that rural care is very important; but all the other experiences they have tend to make cities and big hospitals seem more exciting and more important.

> All experiences tend to shape attitudes—not just the experiences which are designed to change attitudes.

Because of this, teachers must think what kind of attitudes might result from all aspects of the curriculum. For example, they should consider (amongst many other things):

- The proportions of time spent in the field and the classroom.
- Whether the training should be based in a village or a city.
- Whether hospital consultants or PHC workers do the teaching.
- Whether the assessment is competitive.
- Whether teachers are seen as the source of all information, or whether students can rely on their own experience and on books, etc.
- Whether the course generates rivalry between different groups of health workers.

etc., etc.

Within this context—that all of the curriculum will influence attitudes—teachers can do specific things which will help to shape attitudes. These are

- Telling students what attitudes are appropriate (section 11.6).
- Encouraging students to discuss attitudes (section 11.7).
- Providing information and experience (section 11.8).
- Providing 'role models' and examples (section 11.9).
- Using role-play exercises (section 11.10).

Each of these techniques are discussed separately below—though in the actual situation of teaching the techniques should be integrated as far as possible.

11.6 TELLING STUDENTS ABOUT ATTITUDES

Telling students what attitude they should adopt cannot be expected to be enough. However, it is sensible to talk to students about the importance of attitudes and to tell them what attitudes PHC workers should have.

Sometimes students will disagree with the teacher. Sometimes they will agree with the teacher at an intellectual level, but not adopt the new attitude at an emotional level (e.g. they might accept that health workers should be meticulous in following aseptic procedures, but in practice they might be rather careless).

Sometimes the students will agree with and adopt the attitude. This will be most likely when the teacher is respected, liked and admired by the students. It is least likely when the teacher is not respected and when the teacher clearly does not have that attitude himself.

11.7 ENCOURAGING STUDENTS TO DISCUSS ATTITUDES

Discussion of attitudes should be done in groups which are small enough for every student to express his ideas.

The aim of the discussion should be to put each student in a situation where he has to:

- explore what their own attitudes are;
- think about whether these attitudes are appropriate;
- consider alternative attitudes.

An example of how this might be done is given below.

A group of students have been taught where to site pit latrines and how to build them. They have had field experience in these skills. Now the teacher divides the whole group into smaller groups of seven or eight students and asks them to discuss and answer the following questions

'You are responsible for environmental health in your district. You know that in several villages there are no pit latrines and that in the few villages where latrines have been built they are dirty and little used. You decide that you want to improve this situation in one of the villages.

How will you start this task? Call a village meeting? Talk with individuals? Do a survey? Get authority from the District Medical Officer?

What will be your approach? The government policy is that all villages should have pit latrines and so you must build them? In the towns people use latrines so should you? Defaecating in fields is unhealthy so you must use pit latrines instead?

What kind of resistance to pit latrines do you expect?

Will you dig the latrines yourself? Or help the village people to dig them? Or supervise the village people whilst they do the digging? Or leave them a set of plans?"

> After about 30 minutes discussion within the groups, bring the groups together to report what they have decided.
>
> During the report, note down differences between the approaches of the different groups. Note down aspects which reflect the kind of attitude you would like the students to have—and aspects which show undesirable attitudes.
>
> Then tell the students what notes you have made and find out what their reaction is.

In all discussions with students the role of the teacher is mainly to ask questions and to provoke students into thinking for themselves.

11.8 PROVIDING INFORMATION AND EXPERIENCE

Attitudes are partly based on logic and partly on emotions. So if you wish to encourage students to be more eager to communicate knowledge and skills, you can provide factual information which shows why this attitude is desirable. For example, you might tell your students about oral rehydration, how mothers can make up their own rehydration mixtures and how they can give it to their own children. You can quote estimates of the number of deaths in infants which could have been prevented if only mothers had known what to do. All this is the logical information which justifies an attitude of sharing knowledge.

You might also show your students a baby which is severely dehydrated and on a drip in a hospital ward, and explain how this baby's suffering is the result of a health worker's failure to share knowledge.

This second example may be less logical and less intellectually accurate; but it may well have more impact on the students' attitudes than numbers and statistics.

Information and experience can be provided by the teacher sharing his own experience or data which have been collected. But students should also have direct experience in the field by working in communities and meeting other health workers. In this way they can observe the attitudes of health workers and they can also see the consequences of both effective and ineffective health care.

Another source of information is through films, tape-slide programmes, pictures, posters and books.

Sometimes the information or experience will be so dramatic that it will lead directly to attitude changes. At other times the teacher should follow the experience with discussion sessions as outlined in section 11.7. This will review the experience, allow students to share their reactions with each other and explore what consequences can be deduced from the experience.

11.9 PROVIDING ROLE MODELS AND EXAMPLES

The attitudes of teachers and other health workers are amongst the most powerful influences on students' attitudes. The most common link is for students to copy the attitudes and ways of working of teachers and health workers they admire.

Therefore it is important for teachers to provide a 'role model'. A teacher who impressed one of the authors was the Principal of a school for health assistants. One of the tasks of the health assistants was to encourage agriculture in villages and in this way improve nutrition. However, the common local attitude was that digging was menial and undignified. So, many health assistants felt agriculture was not important and was beneath their status. The Principal overcame this attitude by going into the school field with the students, digging irrigation channels himself and joining in the planting and harvesting of crops. He provided an excellent role model and was certainly more effective in shaping favourable attitudes to agriculture and manual work than any lectures or logical arguments.

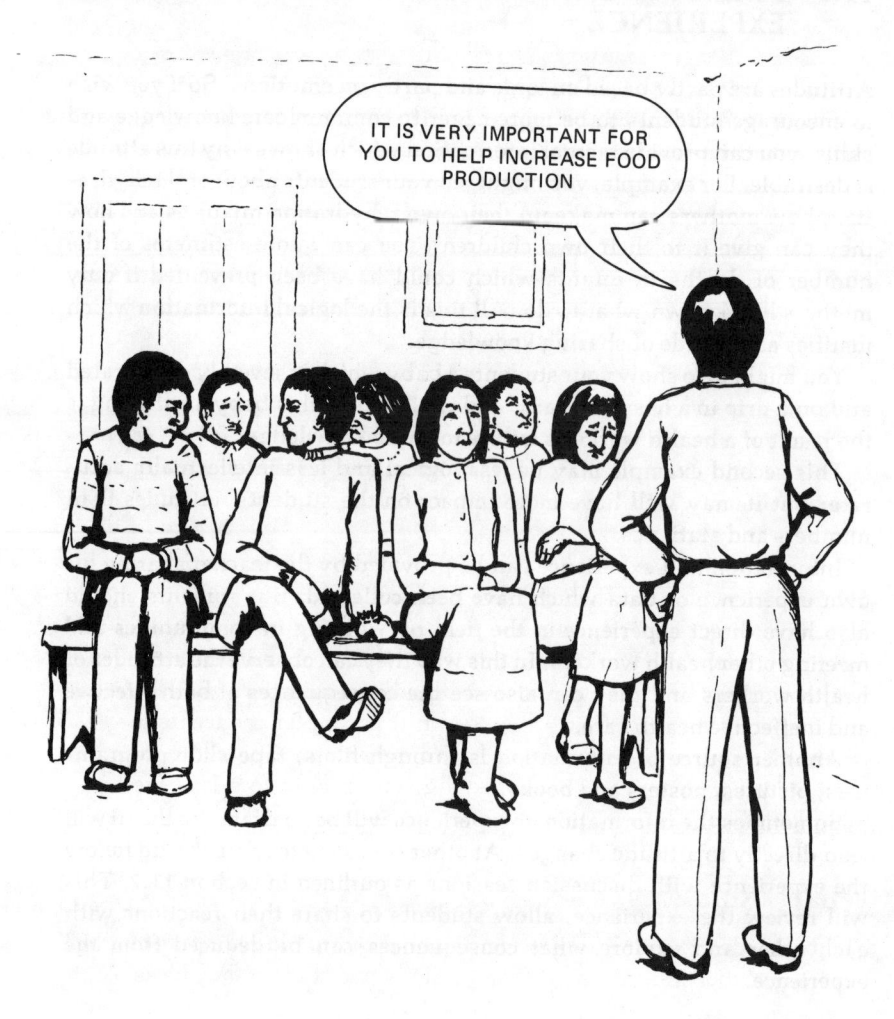

Figure 11.3 Which would be more likely to influence a student's attitudes?

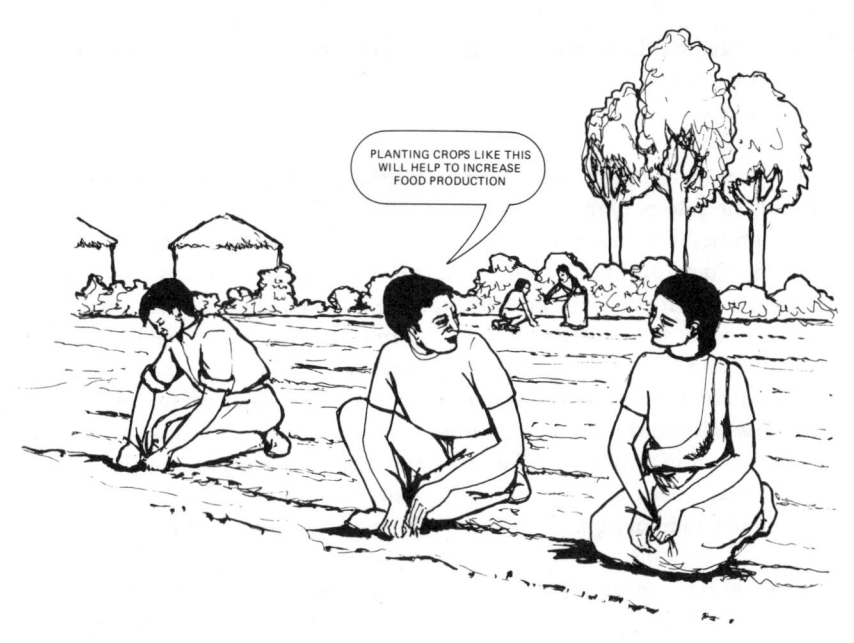

Figure 11.4 Which would be more likely to influence a student's attitudes?

This is a fairly dramatic example. But all teachers have many opportunities to demonstrate their own attitudes in smaller ways. Is the teacher willing to admit that he had made a mistake? Does the teacher give the impression that he knows everything in his field? Does the teacher treat students, colleagues, patients and people living in the community with friendliness and respect? Does the teacher accept poor quality work? All the time, teachers display their own attitudes—often unconsciously. It is therefore important to appoint teachers who do believe in the vital importance of PHC and in the importance of communities developing their own capacity to care for their own health.

Teachers should also spend some time in examining what their own attitudes are, and whether they are appropriate.

Teachers organising field work should also try to make sure that the students come in contact with health workers who will provide the best possible role models.

11.10 USING ROLE-PLAY EXERCISES

Role-play exercises can and should be widely used in training PHC workers. They are useful in teaching communication and decision-making skills as well as attitudes. So in this chapter the technique as a whole is described and examples given for teaching attitudes. In the other chapters on teaching skills, advice is given on how to adapt the basic role-play technique to teach the various skills.

What is Role Play?

The basic idea is that a few students are asked to play the part of other people in a specified situation. For example, one student may be asked to be a village health worker, another will be a mother with a malnourished baby, a third will be the baby's grandmother. The situation could be the health worker visiting the family to explain how the mother could better feed her baby.

This basic situation can be made a little bit more elaborate by telling each of the role players a little bit more about their character or opinions. For example, the grandmother might be told that she is very conservative, has brought up eight children and thinks she knows what food is good for them. The mother might be told that she has had some education and is open to ideas, but is frightened of the grandmother. The health worker might be told that she is rather bossy and unsympathetic—all she knows is the nutritional value of foods and cannot understand that other people may have different ideas or customs.

The situation can also be made more explicit. For example, the health worker may only have 10 min for the visit, the mother's husband may be a farmer who is in debt and has to sell all he grows to pay off the debt, etc., etc.

In general the teacher should define the people and the situation in about as much detail as is given above. More detail will make it very difficult for the students playing the roles to follow all the instructions. Fewer details may leave the students too uncertain about what they should do.

The teacher should explain each of the roles and describe the situation to the class. Then ask the role players to start.

In this case the health worker might greet the mother and grandmother, explain what the visit is about and start to explain about nutrition. The grandmother might interrupt and disagree or the mother might ask for help about how the different foods can be obtained. The group will talk and behave as they imagine the real people would.

The role play may come to a natural end (e.g. the health worker leaves the house) or the teacher may decide that it has gone on long enough for the educational purpose and stop the play.

A variation of the above pattern is to define the roles one day and then ask the students to perform the role play on a later day. This allows time for preparation, but it does need more careful planning by the teacher.

This then is the role play itself. If the role play stops here it provides variety and interest in a teaching situation. But it is hardly a learning experience. To transform the role play from entertainment to purposeful learning, the teacher must prepare the audience and follow the role play with a structured discussion.

What Should the Audience Do?

The audience must be guided in what they should observe. In the role play above they could be:

- Checking the accuracy of the nutritional information provided by the health worker.
- Noting the communication skills of the health worker.
- Interpreting the attitudes of each of the role players.

- Wondering how they would feel if they were the grandmother—or the mother—in that situation.
- Comparing the beliefs about nutrition expressed by the mother/grandmother with the beliefs of people in the students' own villages.

All these things are possible and so the audience must be guided about where they should concentrate their attention. In this case since the purpose of the role play is to develop attitudes, the students should concentrate on the attitudes and feelings of the role players.

This concentration may be helped by having a specially prepared checklist to fill in or a set of questions to answer. This is often useful, but the teacher must balance the potential benefit of the checklists/questions against the effort involved in preparation. A compromise which is often appropriate is to explain what the audience should look for without preparing a written checklist.

Follow-up

At the end of the role play the teacher should lead the discussion. Often this will start with some kind of general question such as 'Well . . . what are your reactions to what you have seen? What did you think of that?'.

The students should then be guided into more specific observations by asking questions such as 'Do you feel that this health worker was sympathetic to the problems of the mother?'.

These observations of attitudes shown in the role play can then be compared with the audience's own attitudes, by asking questions like, 'Do you have the same attitudes as the health worker?'.

The final stage of the discussion might be to debate what attitudes are appropriate. The teacher could ask, 'What would happen if health workers . . .?' or, 'What attitude should health workers have towards . . .?'.

Summarising

There is a lot of value in encouraging students to talk about attitudes, to explore what they believe, to discuss what is appropriate. Yet this discussion can seem rather purposeless and the conclusion may seem rather vague.

So it is important to bring the session to a conclusion by summarising what has been discussed. The main points should be written down on the chalkboard or the students might be asked to spend 4 min writing down their own summaries in their notes.

Review of the Teacher's Role

When using a role play the teacher should:

(i) Decide what the students should learn in the role play exercise (i.e. what attitudes, what skills).

(ii) Devise a fairly simple situation with only 2, 3 or 4 role players and work out an outline for who each person is and what their background/character is.
(iii) Explain to the role players what they should do—and if possible give them time for preparation.
(iv) Explain to the audience what they should look for during the role play.
(v) Lead a purposeful discussion after the role play, bringing out the important features (this should be done mainly by the teacher asking questions rather than by giving answers).
(vi) Make sure that the session is summarised.

11.11 SOME EXAMPLES OF ROLE PLAYS

A number of examples of situations which can form the basis for role plays are given below. This is done to stimulate teachers to develop these according to their own needs and to think of other role plays which may be more appropriate.

(1) A medical assistant is taking a history from a mother whose child has a headache and fever. At that point the medical assistant's supervisor walks in and says, 'I would like to talk to you for a few minutes'.
(This could explore the attitudes of both the health worker and the supervisor to the importance of patients.)
(2) A health worker tries to persuade a mother of 7 children to use contraception. The mother does not want to. (The woman's husband may also be included in this role play.)
(3) A health inspector tries to persuade a group of village headmen that the community should build a well. One of the headmen thinks the government should do the building. Another does not want the well to be built at all. The third agrees with the health inspector.
(4) A health worker is weighing a pregnant lady in an antenatal clinic when the wife of the local chief/politician comes into the clinic and demands that the health worker provides her with penicillin tablets immediately.

These and many, many other situations can be used to provide the basis for learning about the attitudes of other people and developing the students' own attitudes.

11.12 ASSESSING ATTITUDES

It is difficult to find out what a person's attitudes are.
Suppose that you ask a student, 'Do you want to cooperate with other health workers in promoting health care?'. The student may answer 'Yes'. But is this the student's real attitude or is it just the student giving the answer which he thinks you want?

Suppose that you visit a trainee health worker during a period of field work in a health centre. You notice that the trainee follows aseptic techniques carefully. But is this because the trainee's attitude is one of care and concern to maintain aseptic conditions, or is it because the trainee knows that you are watching and would behave quite differently if he was not observed?

So assessing attitudes is difficult and therefore—because the assessment is so uncertain—attitude assessment should not be part of any final examination or count for marks in the overall decision to qualify a student.

Yet this situation is unsatisfactory. We have argued that attitudes are very important—but that we should not assess them in the final examination.

The suggested solution to this problem is

> Attitudes should be assessed during the course

This assessment should be used to give feedback to each individual student. The results should be discussed to find out whether the student agrees with the assessment and whether a change in attitude is appropriate.

What methods can be used to assess attitudes? Psychologists and psychometrists use a wide range of written and visual methods. All these methods require specialised training to develop the attitude scale and the reliability of the attitude measurement is often still open to debate. So attitude questionnaires and written tests are *not* recommended in training PHC workers.

A more practical approach is to observe the way in which students work in the field and deduce from this what the students' attitudes are likely to be.

A rating scale to be completed by a field work supervisor

Attitude to learning
Disinterested, makes little effort ⊢—+—+—+—⊣ Enthusiastic, eager to learn

Response to advice
Doesn't like to be advised, does not follow the advice given ⊢—+—+—+—⊣ Welcomes advice, and follows the advice

Initiative
Does the minimum amount of work possible ⊢—+—+—+—⊣ Undertakes useful work without being asked

Sharing ideas
Gives the minimum amount of information to patients ⊢—+—+—+—⊣ Keen to explain as much as possible about health care to patients

_____

_____

To help this observation—and to reach some consistency between different observers—a rating scale is useful.

Teachers can develop their own rating scale quite simply. The examples given below will give a guide.

Notice that this rating scale does not assess the students' knowledge or skill, but just their approach to the work.

The rating scale is filled in by the supervisor/teacher who puts a cross on the line at any point between the two ends. For example, a student who seems quite interested in learning, sometimes asks the supervisor a question, but perhaps doesn't look up the manuals very often to check his knowledge, would be rated a bit to the right of centre of the scale, e.g.

Attitude to learning

Disinterested, makes little effort ├───┼───┼─X─┼───┤ Enthusiastic, eager to learn

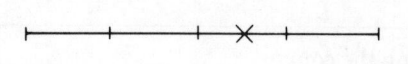

It is comparatively simple to devise rating scales using this technique. And they do help to make rating more objective. However, it is still rather subjective. Should the student described above have the cross marked a little further to the right? Or to the left?

This subjectivity can be reduced by describing each of the intermediate points, e.g.

Response to advice

├───────┼───────┼───────┼───────┤

| Dislikes advice. Defends previous actions. Ignores what is said and continues in just the same way | Neutral reaction to advice. Sometimes follows the advice, but seems reluctant to change | Neutral reaction to advice. Usually tries to follow the advice. Willing to change | Welcomes advice. Follows the advice unquestioningly | Welcomes advice and seeks help when in doubt. Discusses the advice given and is eager to improve |

This development of the rating scale is more difficult to prepare but usually makes it easier to fill in. It also makes it easier to interpret a rating made by another person. The main problem is that it is difficult to anticipate all the possible attitudes and behaviours. For example, in the case above, how would you record a student who always seemed to welcome advice, but who rarely followed the advice given?

In choosing the type of rating scale to be used, consider the amount of time available for preparing the rating scale and remember that its main purpose is to provide feedback to students so that they can become more conscious of their attitudes and develop them so that they will be more effective as PHC workers.

SUMMARY

Attitudes are difficult to define precisely, but are very important as they shape the behaviour of health workers.

Attitudes which are necessary for effective PHC work are to some extent different from the attitudes associated with purely curative care.

Attitudes can be taught by:

- telling students what attitudes are important;
- encouraging students to discuss attitudes;
- providing information and experience;
- providing role models and examples;
- using role-play exercises.

Attitudes can be assessed in the field using rating scales. This assessment should be mainly used to give feedback to the students.

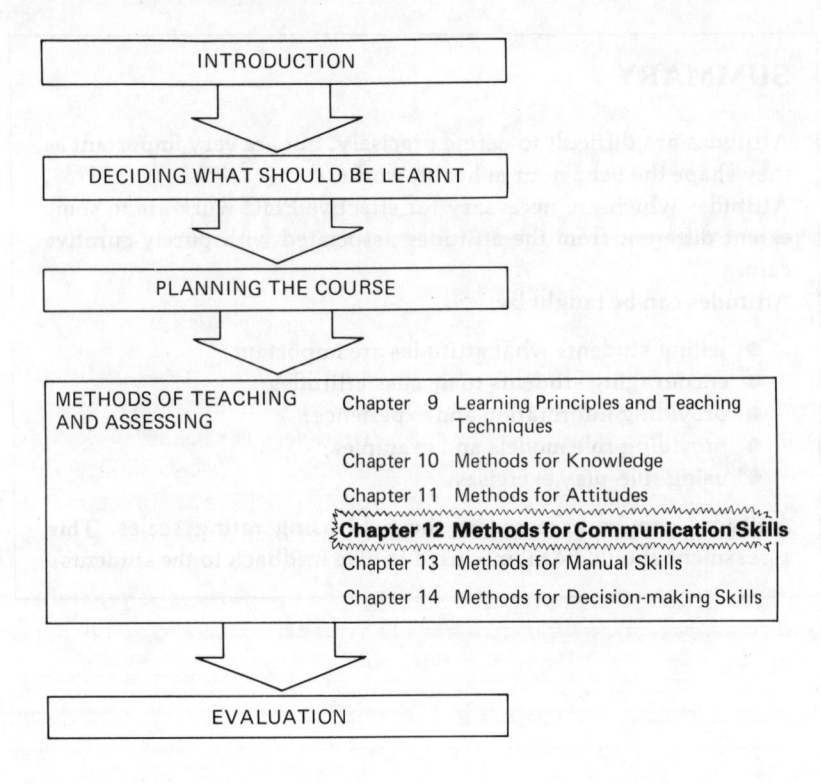

```
                    ┌─────────────────────────┐
                    │      INTRODUCTION       │
                    └─────────────────────────┘
                                │
                                ▼
                    ┌─────────────────────────┐
                    │ DECIDING WHAT SHOULD BE LEARNT │
                    └─────────────────────────┘
                                │
                                ▼
                    ┌─────────────────────────┐
                    │   PLANNING THE COURSE   │
                    └─────────────────────────┘
                                │
                                ▼
```

METHODS OF TEACHING AND ASSESSING	Chapter 9	Learning Principles and Teaching Techniques
	Chapter 10	Methods for Knowledge
	Chapter 11	Methods for Attitudes
	Chapter 12	**Methods for Communication Skills**
	Chapter 13	Methods for Manual Skills
	Chapter 14	Methods for Decision-making Skills

```
                                │
                                ▼
                    ┌─────────────────────────┐
                    │       EVALUATION        │
                    └─────────────────────────┘
```

CONTENTS

12.1	What are Communication Skills?	160
12.2	General Method of Teaching Communication Skills	163
12.3	Analysing Communication Skills	163
12.4	Describing and Demonstrating Communication Skills	164
12.5	Providing Practice in Performing Communication Skills	165
12.6	Group Discussions	166
12.7	Role Play	170
12.8	Field Experience/Interviews	172
12.9	Written Communication—Project Work	173
12.10	Assessing Communication Skills	174

12
Teaching and Assessing Communication Skills

One of the features of Primary Health Care (PHC) that makes it different from the medical care model is the emphasis on communication. Many of the parts of PHC simply cannot take place unless the health workers are effective communicators. Examples of situations where communication is necessary include all aspects of health education, encouraging community participation, developing intersectoral cooperation and sharing knowledge about health so that individual people can take more responsibility for looking after themselves. The emphasis on these areas is comparatively new; however medical care has always been more successful where there has been effective communication between the patient and the doctor or nurse. Therefore

> Communication skills are essential skills in providing health care

This chapter will discuss how these skills can be taught and assessed. But first the skills themselves will be described.

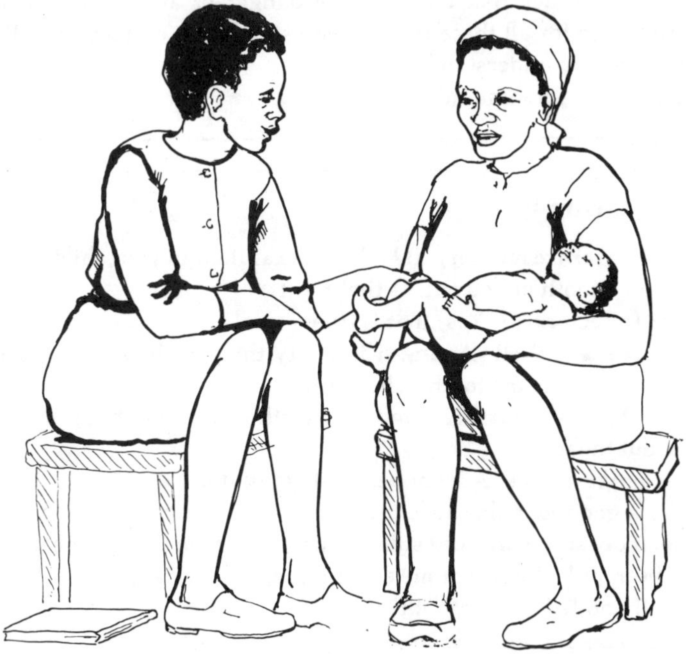

Figure 12.1 'Communication skills are essential skills in providing health care'

12.1 WHAT ARE COMMUNICATION SKILLS?

In the introduction to this chapter we have argued that communication skills are essential. Most health workers and most trainers would probably agree with this conclusion. 'Communication' is a 'good thing'. But what, exactly, are communication skills?

We can start off by saying that they are the skills used when one informs, persuades, explains, tells, listens, makes clear, demonstrates, etc., etc. So, for example, one must teach health workers how to 'explain' as part of their communication skills. But what exactly is involved in 'explaining'? May be this can be illustrated by the following two conversations. Both of the conversations took place in an area where it is common for mothers to extract the teeth of babies who suffer from diarrhoea in the belief that it is 'teething' which causes the diarrhoea. In both conversations a health worker is talking to the mother of a child whose teeth have been pulled out.

Conversation A

Health worker (to mother): I see that your child has had a tooth pulled out. Is that right?

Mother (reluctantly): Yes. That is true.

Health worker: I suppose that you or your mother pulled the tooth out because your child had diarrhoea. Well, this is wrong. It is a bad thing to do. When you pull the tooth out you cause a haemorrhage and the child may lose a lot of blood—possibly so much that the child dies. Another risk factor is that the wound may become infected, cause septicaemia and again the child can die. Yet another risk factor is the danger of an air embolism forming. So for all these reasons you should not extract a child's tooth. Do you understand?

Mother: Yes, I understand.

Conversation B

Health worker (to mother): It looks to me as though your child, Etit, has had a tooth pulled out. Is that right?

Mother (reluctantly): Yes, that is true.

Health worker: Well, Anam, it is a pity that Etit has lost a good tooth. Why was the tooth pulled out?

Mother: He had diarrhoea and new teeth cause diarrhoea, so we take out the tooth.

Health worker: I see. A lot of people do that, don't they? But it isn't really a good idea, because there are a lot of dangers. And in any case, it doesn't work. Etit still has diarrhoea even though the tooth has been pulled out. Let me explain some of the dangers . . . Who actually pulled out the tooth?

Mother: My mother did it.

Health worker: How did she do it?

Mother: Oh, she used a nail and sort of flicked out the tooth . . . just the way we always do it.

Health worker: I expect this hurt your child a lot and probably the gum kept on bleeding. Is that so?

Mother: Yes, it did bleed for quite a bit. But I stopped the bleeding by pressing my finger over the hole.

Health worker: Good. But what had you been doing just before this time?

Mother: I think that I was milking the camels.

Health worker: I suppose that you wouldn't have had a chance to wash your hands after milking?

Mother: No. There is so little water here.

Health worker: Well, Anam, I think you have been lucky, because this time Etit still seems to be quite well. But you took some serious risks.

Sometimes when a tooth is pulled out the child keeps on bleeding and the mother cannot stop the blood flowing. Do you remember that baby in Kengolekerion village who died about 10 days ago?

Mother: Yes. I heard about it.

Health worker: Well, this was the reason. When the baby's tooth was pulled out it just kept bleeding until the baby did not have enough blood left to stay alive.

Another danger is that you can get dirt into the blood. When you were milking the camel your fingers could have been dirty from touching the camel. Then when you pressed your finger against the gum, the dirt from the camel could have got into your child's blood. This sometimes causes very serious illness. Do you know that dirt in the blood can make people very ill?

Mother: Oh yes, I know that. That is why we use clean water to clean cuts when we are cut by a knife or when we work in the field.

Health worker: Yes, that's right. This is just the same kind of thing. You must not let any dirt get in the wound.

So, Anam . . . can you tell me the reasons why pulling out teeth is not a good thing to do?

Mother: Yes. Because pulling out the tooth doesn't stop the diarrhoea and it is dangerous.

Health worker: Yes, that's right. But why is it dangerous?

Mother: Oh! That's because the gum can keep on bleeding till the baby dies and also dirt can get into the wound.

Health worker: That's it. Yes. So I hope you won't want to pull out the teeth from any other babies. Do you think that you could explain this to your friends in the village?

Mother: Yes. I will.

These two conversations illustrate two quite different ways of explaining. The second is obviously much longer and will take far more time. But if it is more effective than the first, surely this time is very well spent.

At this point try reading through the two conversations again and try to identify the good and bad things about each attempt at explanation. Then compare your thoughts with the list below.

Features of the Two Conversations

Conversation A	*Conversation B*
1. Brief and quick	Much longer, but only takes 3 min
2. Related to a real problem which the mother has	Related to a real problem which the mother has
3. Clear and systematic structure to the argument	Clear and systematic structure, but a bit less clear than A
4. Ignores what the mother knows	Finds out the mother's reasons and what the mother already knows
5. The explanation is theoretical and not related to the mother's experience	Relates the explanation to what the mother already knows and does
6. Does *not* find out whether the mother has understood. (The question 'do you understand?' is a waste of time because very few people will actually say 'No', even when they don't understand)	Finds out whether the mother has understood. This is done by asking the mother to explain and following up the first answer to make sure that she knows what the dangers are
7. Uses unfamiliar words, e.g. haemorrhage, risk factor, infected, septicaemia, air embolism	Uses words which the mother herself uses
8. Blames or condemns the mother's actions	Avoids blaming
9. Impersonal	Uses Anam's name and more personal tone
10. A quick clear explanation to a trained nurse, but not suitable for Anam	A much better explanation for Anam

---

One point that cannot be illustrated in print is the tone of voice. This can either help explanation or can be threatening. For example, try saying to yourself 'Is that right?' in different ways. Emphasise each word in turn. Imagine how you would say it if you didn't believe what you had just heard, or if you thought that what you had just heard was true but very wicked. The tone of voice can be all important.

The point of all the above is to show that

> effective explanation is much more than just telling

The list of points begins to define what is meant by 'explaining'. This list will, in turn, guide a teacher in what students should learn when they are learning to explain.

12.2 THE GENERAL METHOD OF TEACHING COMMUNICATION SKILLS

The overall pattern of teaching communication skills is as follows.

- Analysing each of the communication skills (section 12.3).
- Describing and demonstrating each of the communication skills to the learners (section 12.4).
- Providing practice so that every one of the learners practises the skills and gets feedback on the quality of the performance (sections 12.5–12.9).
- Assessing whether full competence has been achieved (section 12.10).

Each of these stages will be explained in more detail in the sections below.

12.3 ANALYSING COMMUNICATION SKILLS

It would be impossible to teach the skills of nursing care without knowing what those skills were. In the same way, communication skills cannot be taught unless you first analyse what communication skills are needed.

This analysis can be started by thinking about when the health worker needs to communicate. For example, it might be when the health worker:

- explains to a mother why her baby should be immunised;
- persuades a family to use a pit latrine;
- asks a village meeting to choose their village health worker;
- finds out why a mother does not want to breastfeed her baby;
- discusses with an agricultural adviser how nutrition can be improved in a village;
- explains to a patient what anaemia is and how it can be prevented;
- writes to request that the health centre roof is repaired.

The next stage of the analysis is to separate the facts or information from the skills of communication. For example, think about the situation when a health worker explains to a mother that her baby needs to be immunised. There will be some facts—what the word immunisation means, what the mother will have to do, the benefits of immunisation, etc. But there are also the skills involved in explaining—use of appropriate words which the mother will understand, arranging the facts in a logical order, asking the mother questions to find out whether she understands, etc., etc.

These are the skills which need to be taught.

Another method which can help in analysing communication skills is to ask the question

> 'What is good (or bad) about that communication?'

or a slightly different question

> 'How would one do that communication well?'

The answers to these questions will help to build up a picture of the communication skills to be taught. This list of skills is therefore the set of objectives for the teaching of communication skills.

12.4 DESCRIBING AND DEMONSTRATING COMMUNICATION SKILLS

Describing and demonstrating communication skills is done in much the same way as describing or demonstrating any other skills.
The skills can be described by:

- the teacher telling the learners how to do the skill;
- providing manuals or handouts in which the skills are described.

This description will tend to be rather meaningless in itself and so must be accompanied by demonstration of the skills. This can be done by:

- The teacher performing the skill, e.g. by communicating with either a real patient or with one of the learners who acts the role of the patient.
- The teacher arranging for the students to see a health worker performing the skill. (This may either be in the field, or the health worker may be asked to come to the teaching session.)
- Using videotapes or films or even tape recordings of people performing communication skills. For many teachers this will not be feasible. But those teachers who have any of these facilities should use them. Film and videotape especially are very helpful. The powerful advantages of these techniques are that they bring the field situation into a classroom without all the bother of arranging transport or meetings. They also allow the teacher to show exactly the same communication several times to illustrate a particular point.

Whichever form of demonstration is used, the learners should not be just passive observers. They should be given specific points to look for and the demonstration should be reviewed after it is completed. For example, the teacher might give the students the following questions to answer whilst watching a health inspector persuading a family to use a pit latrine.

Observation checklists like this make the demonstration so much more valuable. They focus the students' attention on what the teacher wants them to see. They also provide an excellent framework for discussion after the demonstration. They can be used whether the demonstration is in the field, in the classroom or on film/videotape.

OBSERVATION OF COMMUNICATION SKILLS

Facts
What were the main reasons given by the Health Inspector?
_____
_____

Manner
Was the H.I.

friendly ├──────┼──────┼──────┤ bossy

rude ├──────┼──────┼──────┤ polite

sympathetic to ├──────┼──────┼──────┤ unsympathetic
problems of family

Language
Which words did the H.I. use which the family might not understand?
_____

Techniques	Yes	No
Did the H.I. reach an agreement with the family?	——	——
Did the H.I. find any reasons which the family already had for using the pit latrine?	——	——
Was the structure of the argument clear?	——	——
Did the H.I. use any visual methods to help in the explanation?	——	——
Success		
Did the H.I. succeed in persuading the family to use the pit latrine?	——	——

What were the reasons for his success or lack of success?
_____
_____

12.5 PROVIDING PRACTICE IN PERFORMING COMMUNICATION SKILLS

This is the really crucial stage in teaching communication skills. It is also the most difficult to organise. Is it worth the inevitable effort? Well, imagine that you have to fly in an aeroplane to another country. When you have sat down in the aeroplane, they announce, 'Inshallah Airways welcome you aboard. Your pilot is Captain X. He has just finished his pilot training which has involved listening to lectures on how to fly aeroplanes and he has attended many hours of demonstration. He hasn't yet actually touched the controls of any aircraft or flown. But he wrote excellent essays on the theory of flight and scored 86% on a multiple choice question paper. We are sure you will be glad to know that his knowledge is so up-to-date'.

Providing practice is essential. But it is difficult to arrange, because every student must have the practice and they must have someone to communicate with when they are practising.

The methods which are commonly used to provide practice in communication skills include:

Group discussions (section 12.6)
Role play (section 12.7)
Field experience/interviews (section 12.8)
Written exercises (section 12.9)

12.6 GROUP DISCUSSIONS

Group discussions can and should be widely used in training health workers. They can be used to discuss the application of facts or principles in problem-solving situations. Thus the discussions can help the learning of facts and principles. In chapter 14, two highly structured methods of holding group discussions (brain-storming and snowballing) are described as a way of developing decision-making skills. In the same chapter, simulations, case histories and patient-management problems all provide a context in which group discussions should take place. Discussions are also advocated as a way of developing attitudes (section 11.7). In all these situations, the students' communication skills can also be developed.

Thus, group discussions can be widely used to help achieve a wide range of objectives. Why are group discussions so widely useful? The essential difference between group discussions and formal lectures or films, is that the students are actively involved in applying ideas, thinking of solutions and expressing their thought. It is this participation which makes group discussions effective as a teaching method. So it is clear that one of the jobs of the teacher is to make sure that all of the students do take an active part.

Sometimes discussions can seem rather purposeless or confused. Therefore the teacher should aim to keep the debate to the point and provide a structure to the discussion.

Discussions will be more helpful if the atmosphere is relaxed and supportive—an atmosphere in which students can feel confident to express their ideas.

The active involvement of students, clarity of structure and informal atmosphere can be achieved if teachers use the following techniques.

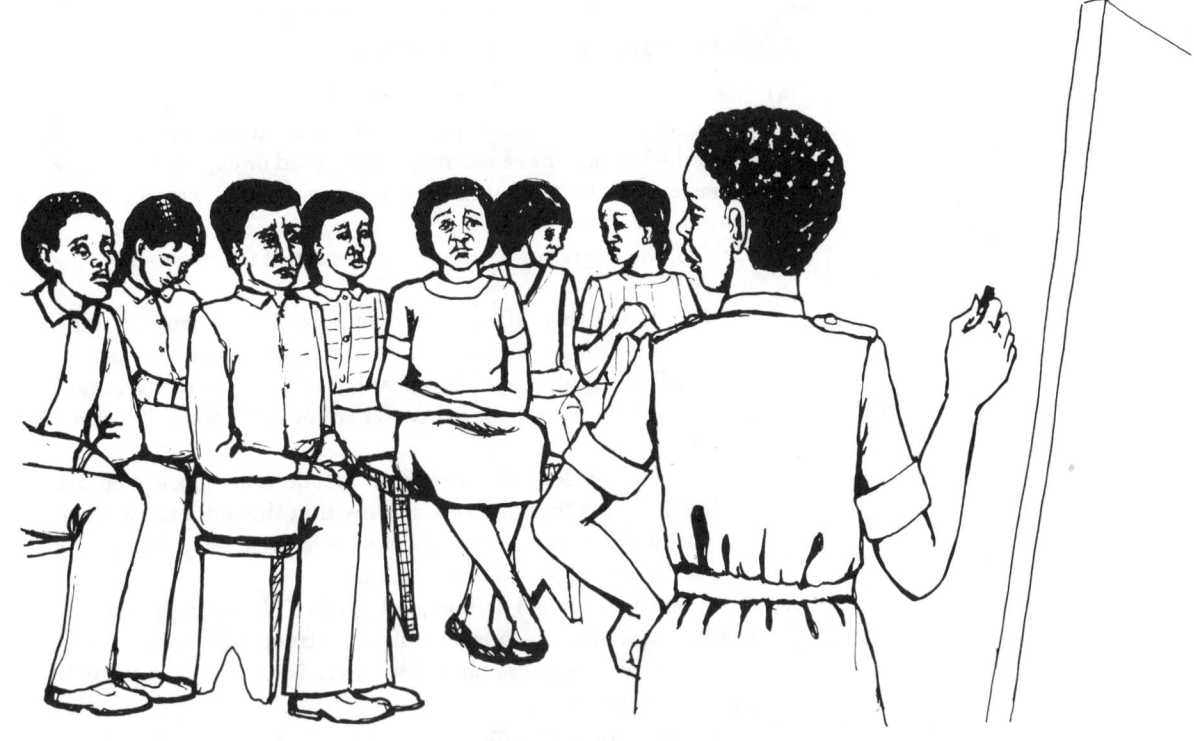

Figure 12.2 'The essential difference between lectures and group discussion is that the students are actively involved'

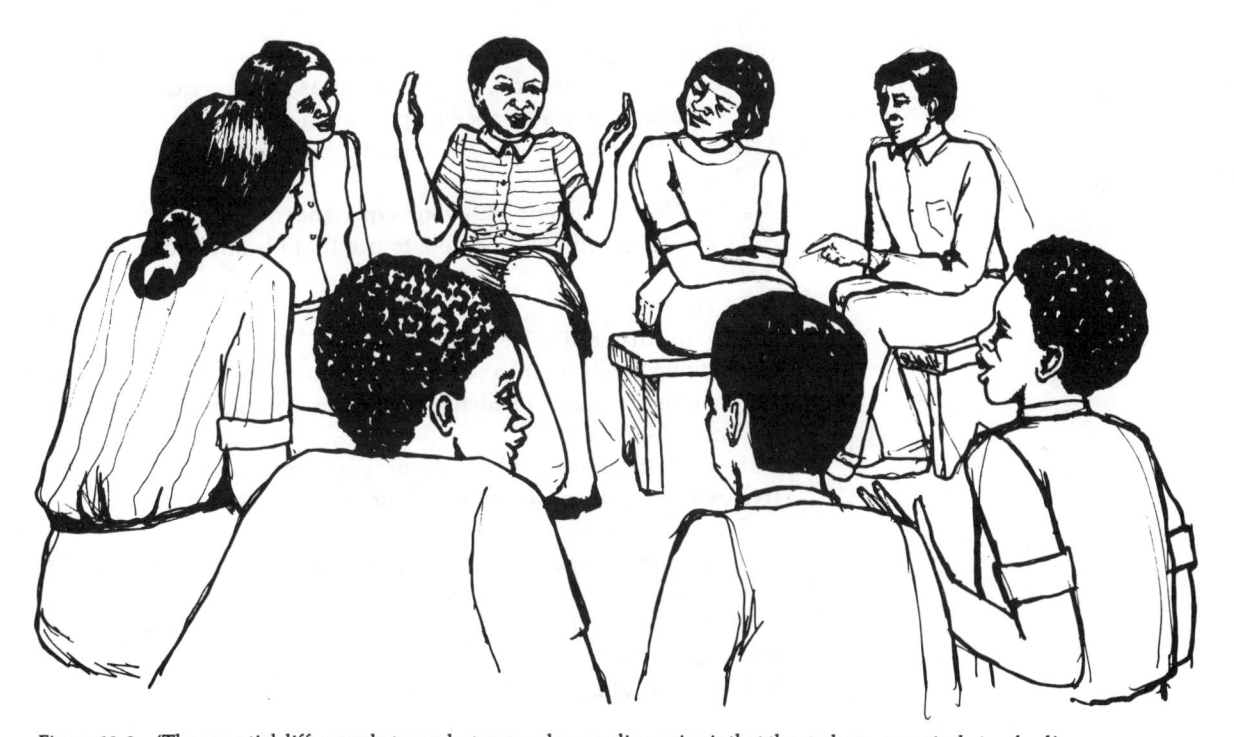

Figure 12.3 'The essential difference between lectures and group discussion is that the students are actively involved'

A Method for Group Discussions

(a) Set the objectives of the sessions (either independently or in discussion with the learners) so that what is to be learnt involves what the learners have recently heard, read or experienced. The essence is to *apply* what has already been partially learnt rather than to cover new ground.

(b) Control the degree of participation of each of the members of the group.

Make sure that all members do participate and that no members dominate the discussion. This is because the exercise of actually formulating opinions and putting them into words is a powerful learning experience. Therefore all should have this experience.

This can be done by directing questions to those who are taking part less than the rest and inviting the more talkative to wait until the others have had a chance to speak. Much depends on the manner in which this is done.

(c) Set a reasonably well defined end-point. This will help to make the discussion more purposeful and structured, so that it is easier for the learners to relate what is being said to their previous knowledge.

This can be done by asking for:
  (i) a list of recommendations;
  (ii) a list of advantages and disadvantages;
  (iii) a decision;
  (iv) appointing one of the learners as a secretary to note down the major points on a board or chart as they are made.
  (The secretary may need help in doing this.)

(d) Maintain the relevance of the discussion by asking questions such as:
  'Is that idea consistent with your experience?'
  'Do you think you will be able to use that idea in your future work?'
  etc., etc.

(e) Clarify the discussion by:
  (i) asking one learner to summarise what another has said;
  (ii) asking learners to identify whether comments are facts or opinions;
  (iii) where clear errors of fact occur, correcting these;
  (iv) referring to the 'secretary's' summary of points made from time to time;
  (v) keeping comments on the main theme of the discussion.

(f) Preparing material for discussion in advance.

This may involve preparing sheets of data, or reference material for the learners to discuss.

It will certainly involve preparing for yourself a list of the

> major points which you feel should be covered and generally being familiar with relevant facts and commonly held opinions.
> (g) Preparing the environment.
>
> All participants in the discussion should be able to see everyone else's face and be close enough to hear each other comfortably.
>
> The environment should also be friendly and relaxed.
>
> If students do not know each other they should be introduced.
>
> The mood should be reasonably lighthearted yet purposeful.
>
> There should be no fear of exposing ignorance.
> (h) The leader should say rather little.
>
> The style of asking questions is vital.
>
> Questions such as, 'Well, what do you think about that?' can be so open-ended that a nervous student will be intimidated. So it may be better to start with a more closed question such as, 'Do you agree with what has just been said?' and then follow this up with, 'Why do you (not) agree?'. The simple question 'Why?' can be very effective in encouraging confident students to clarify what they have said. It can be terrifying to more nervous students.
>
> Above all the Discussion Leader must not give a lecture.

All of the above depends on the discussion taking place in reasonably small groups. Ideally these should consist of 5–9 students, though discussions can be successful with groups of up to about 20 students. The obvious problem with this is that in many training programmes there are large class sizes. To overcome this problem, teachers can:

(a) Use student-led discussion groups. There is no reason why the teacher has to be present in the discussion. When discussions are student-led, the teacher can help by providing some initial training in leading discussion groups, (this can be a very useful skill for a health worker, and so should probably be taught anyway), and by helping set reasonably precise targets for the discussion.
(b) Use discussions within a lecture. This can be done by setting short discussion topics once or twice within a 1-hour presentation. The students can be organised into small groups and briefly report their conclusions within the overall framework of the 'lecture'.

Topics for a discussion session should aim to:

(i) help the students to apply principles or facts that have recently been learnt;
(ii) draw out the experience or attitudes of students.

There are of course very many topics which would be suitable for discussion. A few suggestions are given below.

(1) How would you find out whether hookworm caused serious problems in a health district?

(2) What is the most cost-effective way of reducing the incidence of malaria in this area?
(3) What are the local beliefs or traditions which encourage a healthy life style?
(4) What arguments are likely to be most effective in persuading mothers to breast-feed their babies?

etc., etc.

12.7 ROLE PLAY

The general technique of role play is described in section 11.10. There it is discussed as a method of teaching attitudes. Section 14.12 discusses role play as a way of teaching decision-making skills. Role play is also useful in developing communication skills. In fact many examples of role play will be useful in all these three areas. This section concentrates on describing the ways in which role play can be used to develop communication skills.

In any role play, students will take the role of various people and will talk to each other in some way. Clearly these students who are acting the roles will get practice in communicating.

The students who observe the role play can also learn about communication. This will happen if they critically observe what is good—and what is bad—about the communication they are watching. This critical observation can be guided by the use of checklists such as the one below.

Communication Checklist

Are appropriate visual methods used?
Is the communication brief?
Is the communication unhurried?
Are the facts accurate?
Is the argument logical and clearly structured?
Is enough detail provided?
Are familiar words used?
Is the sentence structure simple?
Is the other person greeted?
Is the other person spoken to by name?
Is the other person's existing knowledge explored?
Are the other person's beliefs respected?
Is credit given for appropriate actions?
Is blame and condemnation avoided?
Is concern shown for the other person's problems?

Is the explanation based on the other person's previous experience?
Does any solution offered actually solve the problem as seen by the other person?

Is the person asked to apply information?
Is the other person's knowledge/understanding tested?

The checklist above is not intended as anything more than a starting point for teachers to develop better and more locally appropriate checklists of their own.

The observation during the role play should then form the basis of a detailed discussion of what could have been done better and how it could have been done, what was done well and why it was good. It is not unusual to have a very profitable discussion for half an hour following a five-minute role play.

Role-play topics are fairly easy to think of. They should normally be based on the day-to-day communications that health workers are involved in. So at least some of the following could be used in many training programmes:

(i) A health worker explains to a mother why and how she can treat her young child with sugar and salt solution when the child has diarrhoea.
(ii) A health worker tries to persuade a patient that an injection is not necessary for a cold.
(iii) A health worker explains to a mother why she should come back for the third DPT injection.
(iv) A health worker explains to a traditional birth attendant how to cut the umbilical cord.
(v) A health worker tries to persuade a village health committee that wells in the village should be better protected.
(vi) A health worker tries to persuade a village health committee to build pit latrines (or to use existing pit latrines).
(vii) A health worker tries to persuade the local school teacher to include more nutrition in the school curiculum.
etc., etc.

Organising role play can be a problem. Ideally there should be 2, 3 or 4 'actors' watched by 5 or 6 students. This size of group gives all students fairly frequent practice in communicating. However, in most training programmes there are rather more than 10 or so students. This means that several teachers will be needed to conduct the role plays—which is often not feasible. An alternative is to run the first few role plays with the whole group of students. Then divide the whole group into smaller groups which can conduct their own role-play exercise. In this situation, the teacher has a management role. The teacher's job is to prepare for the role play by defining the situation and the roles. The teacher should also prepare checklists to help the students to observe the role play critically. During the role play itself, the teacher should move from one group to another ensuring that the work is being done purposefully and possibly guiding the feedback. At the end of the role-play session, the teacher may summarise the key points from what has been observed.

The point of role play is not to replace practice in the real world; it is to prepare students and give them experience in an artificial situation. The point of this is that when the students start to get real experience in the field, they will have had some practice and they will have a basis for criticising (and therefore improving) their standard of communicating.

12.8 FIELD EXPERIENCE/INTERVIEWS

When students have had experience within the training institutions, they should practise communicating in the field under supervision.

This will mean doing the work of a health worker with an experienced supervisor providing detailed and frequent feedback about the quality of the communication. Often this ideal is not possible so an alternative is for other students to provide this feedback.

Whether the feedback is given by students or supervisors the quality and value of this feedback can be increased by using checklists or rating scales.

One of the commonest situations where communication takes place is when a health worker is interviewing a patient or taking a history. An example of a rating scale for this situation is given below as a starting point for teachers to develop their own guides. Note that in this rating scale, the categories 'done well' and 'done poorly' will need to be defined in some detail so that students or supervisors have a clear guide about the standards required.

An Interview/History-taking Rating Scale

	Done well	Done poorly	Not done	Not applicable
The information collected				
Chief complaint				
History of present illness				
Past history of illness				
Family history of illness				
Patient's social history				
Effect of illness on patient and family				
Manner of collecting information				
Follows a logical sequence				
Responds to leads from the patient				
Allows patient to express his concerns				
Uses both open-ended and closed questions				
Uses an appropriate level of language				
Summarises information and allows patient to correct errors				
Establishing a relationship				
Appears friendly and welcoming				
Greets patient and introduces himself				
Uses the patient's name				
Shows concern for the patient				
Uses appropriate gestures and body posture				

Rating scales like the one above should be prepared to suit the local culture. The rating scales should be given to students and discussed with them as a way of describing what is meant by good communication in health care. The completed rating scales should be passed on to the student after the interview as a record and as a basis for improving performance.

Where it is possible, video-tapes are extremely helpful in developing communication skills as they show the student what really happened. Sometimes this can be very surprising to the student who may have been quite unaware of certain mistakes. Although video-tapes are very useful, teachers who do not have access to this kind of equipment should not be discouraged from using role plays. They can still privde very valuable feedback through comments and rating scales or checklists.

12.9 WRITTEN COMMUNICATION—PROJECT WORK

The emphasis above has been on spoken communication. This is appropriate as most of the time health workers will communicate in this way. Yet there are times when written communication is important. For example, health workers may need to write letters to request equipment or other supplies, to present reports of their work or to record specific cases.

To prepare for these kinds of tasks, health workers should be trained in written communication.

This does not mean that students should be asked to write essays or to prepare 'Brief notes on the diagnosis and treatment of Leprosy'. The students will rarely have to do this kind of thing in their professional career, so there seems little point in learning how to do it during the training. Instead, the aim should be to give students practice in the kinds of communication which they will have to do later. Three examples of possible activities are given below. Clearly these will have to be adapted quite substantially to match the requirements of the cadre of health worker being trained.

(1) A group of students is asked to survey a community. They are then asked to prepare a report on the priorities for action which is to be submitted to the community's health committee (or the district health officer).
(2) Each student is asked to imagine that he or she is responsible for a dispensary or a small health centre. The refrigerator is not working *or* the supply of one of the vaccines has run out *or* there is a shortage of a particular drug. (Many other examples could be devised.) The first request to the health worker's supervisor has not been answered. The students are now asked to write a second letter presenting a strong case explaining why action is needed.
(3) Each student is asked to imagine that he or she is a health inspector. They have found that a shop selling meat is not obeying the local regulations. Their task is to write to the shop keeper. (This can be adapted by saying that the shop keeper has ignored a previous letter.)

The role of the teacher in these exercises is first of all to develop realistic situations where written communication is needed. Secondly, some explanation will be needed about the kind of communication which is required and how the communication can be written effectively. The third and absolutely crucial role is to read carefully what each student has written and give detailed feedback about how the writing can be improved. (Giving a mark out of 10 does not guide the student about improvements, only about the overall standard.)

Teachers should not ignore the use of numbers and data in communication. Many health workers will be more effective if they can present numbers effectively by using simple graphs, charts and tables.

12.10 ASSESSING COMMUNICATION SKILLS

Since communication is so important in PHC, communication skills must be assessed.

The general principles of assessment (outlined in chapter 8) require that assessment is valid. This means that the assessment should test those skills which really will be used by the health worker after qualification. This means that the conventional essay examination, multiple-choice questions and even the oral examination are all useless in assessing the communication skills used in health care. This is because health workers are not asked to write essays in their day-to-day work, nor do they answer multiple-choice questions. On the surface, an oral examination does seem to test communication skills—after all the student does have to speak to the examiner. Yet the situation is totally different from the field. The relationship between a student and an examiner is fundamentally different from the relationship between health worker and patient or client. The purpose of the communication is quite different. The student is trying to show how much he knows and a health worker who behaves like this would inevitably be ineffective. The tension and anxiety associated with examinations makes the atmosphere different and of course the examiners will expect quite a different level of use of language. So for all these reasons—whatever other merits they may have—oral examinations cannot effectively test communication skills.

Assessment in the Field

The ideal—as in testing any other skill—is to observe the student working in the field doing the work for which he or she has been trained. This ensures that the assessment is valid. This approach does present serious practical difficulties. These include the problems of arranging for students to have the appropriate field experience, arranging to visit the students whilst they are working and making a reliable assessment of the skill.

These difficulties can sometimes be overcome where there is close co-operation between service staff and the training institution. When this happens, the service staff can often make the assessments. The reliability of their assessments can be increased if checklists or rating scales are used and the service staff are trained in using them. (See the communication checklists in sections 12.7 and 12.8. Also checklists and rating scales in section 13.6c.)

Assessments in the Training Institution

Whilst assessment in the field is ideal, it is often so difficult to organise and so difficult to obtain a uniform standard of marking (i.e. the reliability is low) that field assessment may be impossible or else used as only one part of the whole assessment scheme.

Within the institution, communication skills can be assessed by adapting the teaching methods so that they are used for assessment. The group discussions are of little value in this respect, but adapted role plays and written communications can be used.

Written Communication

The written communications can be assessed in much the same way as any other form of written examination. Points to notice are:

- The examination should allow students sufficient time. In the field, health workers will not need to prepare reports or write letters as part of a race!
- The examination questions themselves may need to be quite long in order to explain what is required of the student. Teachers should not be worried by this. It is far better to write a long clear question than a short ambiguous one.
- It will often be sensible to allow students to refer to manuals or their notes during the examination. This will make the situation more like work in the field where manuals and notes should be used.
- Written communication need not be assessed in an examination environment. Instead students can be asked to prepare projects or specific reports, etc. These can be prepared in the student's free time and then handed in for marking.

Verbal Communication

All the above refers to assessing skills in written communication. But far more important are the skills of verbal communication. These can be assessed by simulating situations in which the student takes the role of a health worker and communicates with a patient, a member of the public or a client. A practical way of organising an examination which does this is called the Objective Structured Practical Examination (OSPE). This is described in section 8.7 of chapter 8.

SUMMARY

- Communication skills are essential skills in providing health care.
- Communication is much, much more than telling. It involves listening, asking, explaining, persuading.
- Communication skills should be analysed, then described and demonstrated.
- Every student should practise communication skills in discussion, role play, field experience and written exercises.
- Skills in communication cannot be assessed in MCQ, essay or oral examinations. Instead, use realistic situations and assist observation with checklists and rating scales. An OSPE is one situation where this can be done.

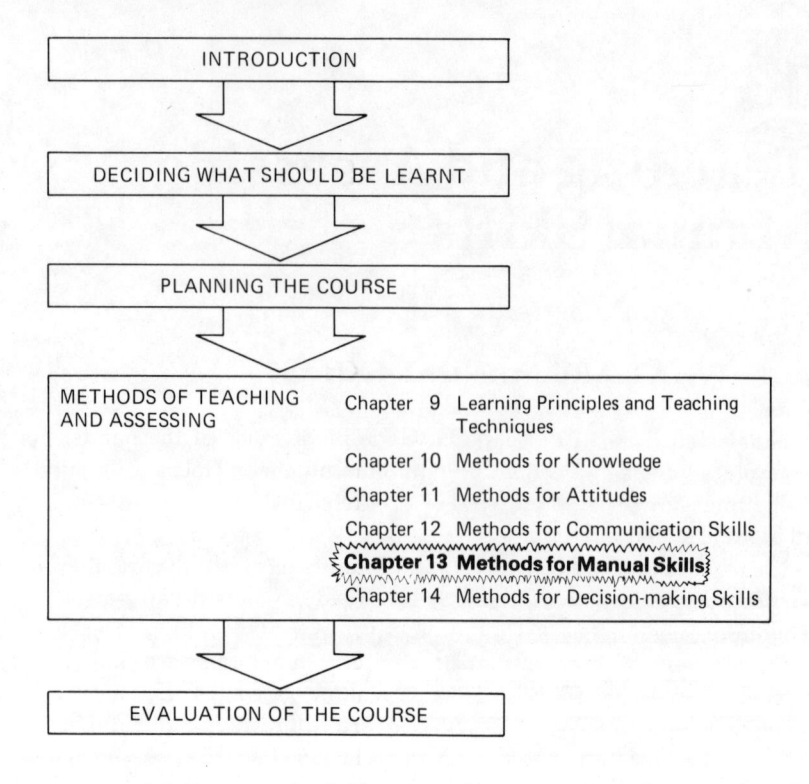

```
        ┌─────────────────────────────┐
        │        INTRODUCTION         │
        └─────────────────────────────┘
                      ▼
        ┌─────────────────────────────┐
        │ DECIDING WHAT SHOULD BE LEARNT │
        └─────────────────────────────┘
                      ▼
        ┌─────────────────────────────┐
        │     PLANNING THE COURSE     │
        └─────────────────────────────┘
                      ▼
┌──────────────────────────────────────────────────────┐
│ METHODS OF TEACHING   Chapter  9  Learning Principles and Teaching
│ AND ASSESSING                    Techniques
│                       Chapter 10  Methods for Knowledge
│                       Chapter 11  Methods for Attitudes
│                       Chapter 12  Methods for Communication Skills
│                       Chapter 13  Methods for Manual Skills
│                       Chapter 14  Methods for Decision-making Skills
└──────────────────────────────────────────────────────┘
                      ▼
        ┌─────────────────────────────┐
        │   EVALUATION OF THE COURSE  │
        └─────────────────────────────┘
```

CONTENTS

13.1	What are Manual Skills?	179
13.2	General Methods for Teaching Manual Skills	180
13.3	Deciding what Skills should be Learnt	180
13.4	Describing and Demonstrating the Manual Skill	181
13.5	Providing Initial Experience in Each Skill: (a) Providing Equipment, Apparatus and Patients—Simulation; (b) Providing enough Time; (c) Providing Detailed Guidance and Feedback—Practice in Pairs, Supervision	182
13.6	Arranging for further Experience: (a) Providing enough Time; (b) Finding suitable Places; (c) Making Clear what Needs to be Learnt—Procedure Book, Checklists, Rating Scales; (d) Achieving Co-operation with Health Service Staff; (e) Providing Appropriate Feedback; (f) Organising a Roster;	186
13.7	Assessing whether Students Have Learnt the Manual Skills	193

13
Teaching and Assessing Manual Skills

13.1 WHAT ARE MANUAL SKILLS?

Manual skills are all those skills which involve use of the hands. For example, giving an injection, palpating an abdomen, focusing a microscope, measuring blood pressure (BP), preparing a blood slide, etc., are all manual skills.

Clearly manual skills are a very important part of health care, they are carried out regularly and frequently by all cadres of health care personnel. Therefore they must be learnt thoroughly.

Quite often the manual skill is part of a more complex skill which involves communication and decision making as well. For example, the whole process of measuring blood pressure will involve explaining to the patient what is going on and making decisions about what action to take following the BP measurement. However this chapter concentrates primarily on the manual aspects of these more complex skills.

Several other words are used to describe these kinds of skills. Psychologists and some educators refer to 'psychomotor skills'. These are the skills which require co-ordination between the brain and the body. Essentially they are the same thing as manual skills. The advantage of using the word 'manual' is that it is shorter and probably more familiar than the rather more precise but longer word 'psychomotor'.

Another word commonly used is 'practical'. This is a slightly unsatisfactory word as it is rather vague. All sorts of skills are practical. For example, the skill of planning health care is 'practical' but it involves very little physical activity. Therefore this book will refer consistently to manual skills.

There is a difference between knowing how to do something and actually being able to do it. For example, many men will know how to thread a needle. (You lick the thread to form a point, then you move the point of the thread through the hole in the needle.) But these same men may not be able to actually thread the needle. They may take a long time or else fail altogether. So they 'know how' but they are not able to do it.

The aim of teaching manual skills is to help the student to be able to *do* the skills, not just know how to do them.

Similarly, the purpose of assessing manual skills is to find out whether students can *do* the skills, not whether they can describe the skills.

13.2 GENERAL METHODS OF TEACHING MANUAL SKILLS

The role of the teacher in teaching manual skills is:

- To decide which manual skills need to be learnt, and to analyse what each of these skills involves (section 13.3).
- To describe and demonstrate each of the skills (section 13.4).
- To arrange for every student to perform each skill (section 13.5).
- To arrange for every student to practise each skill until a satisfactory standard has been reached (section 13.6).
- To assess whether each skill has been learnt to a sufficient standard (section 13.7).

Each of these stages is described in the sections below.

13.3 DECIDING WHAT SKILLS SHOULD BE LEARNT

The earlier chapters of this book have described how to prepare a list of tasks. These will involve communication and decision-making skills as well as the manual skills. Therefore each teacher should review his list of tasks and select those tasks or parts of tasks which are mainly manual.

This list of manual tasks will be specific to the cadre of health worker being trained and to the country where the health workers will be employed. However, some suggestions of manual skills which are commonly performed by health workers are given in chapter 5 and in Appendix 2. These lists can be used as a guide to help teachers prepare their own lists of tasks involving manual skills.

The next stage is to analyse each of the tasks, in order to identify the stages and the sequence in which these tasks are performed. This process is described in chapter 6.

It is a good idea at this time to note down for each stage (or sub-task) any special points about how it can be done well or about mistakes which are commonly made.

An example is given below of a list of steps or stages involved in giving an intramuscular injection in the upper outer quadrant of the buttock. (Notice that this analysis ignores all the communication aspects and all the preparation.)

An Analysis of the Steps in Giving an Intramuscular Injection

Assemble the syringe using sterile technique (previously learned).
Draw up the medicine to be injected.
Remove air (point the needle upwards and gently press the plunger).
Identify and clean the upper outer quarter of the buttock.
Insert the needle rapidly at the correct angle.

> Check that the needle is not in a blood vessel by slightly withdrawing the plunger.
> Inject the medicine.
> Withdraw the needle and syringe.
> Rub over the area rapidly.
> Place the syringe and needle in the discarding dish.

This analysis will involve a lot of work. However, the benefits are enormous since this analysis forms the basis of what will be taught, it can be given to students as a permanent reference, it can guide service personnel in teaching the students and it can form the basis of checklists used in assessing students.

A further point is that the teacher can refer to manuals or procedure books where they may well find that this sort of analysis has already been done for them. So it may only be necessary to copy what has already been written or to adapt it slightly to suit local circumstances.

13.4 DESCRIBING AND DEMONSTRATING THE MANUAL SKILL

The students must be told what manual skills they should learn. This is done by both describing and by demonstrating the skill.

The description should normally be both written and verbal (provided the health workers are literate). The written description can either be something which is prepared by the teacher (i.e. the task analysis referred to in section 13.3) or a page in a manual. It is very desirable for students to have a permanent record describing every skill which they are to learn. This will be valuable both during training and after qualification as a reference.

The verbal description is most usefully done at the same time as the skill is demonstrated.

What are the qualities of a good demonstration—one from which students can actually learn the steps of a procedure?

- A demonstration should be visible to all students. This obvious fact is often ignored—especially in clinics and around a patient's bed in a ward. Sometimes it is necessary to divide the group of students and repeat the demonstration several times.
- A demonstration must be as near as possible to the real thing—preferably, the real thing itself. A performance full of objects substituting for other objects is highly confusing for students. Where substitutes are necessary, there must be no doubt what they represent.
- When demonstrating the injection as above, the teacher will need a real syringe, an actual bottle of the medicine to be injected (though the medicine could be water), alcohol and a swab for cleaning the

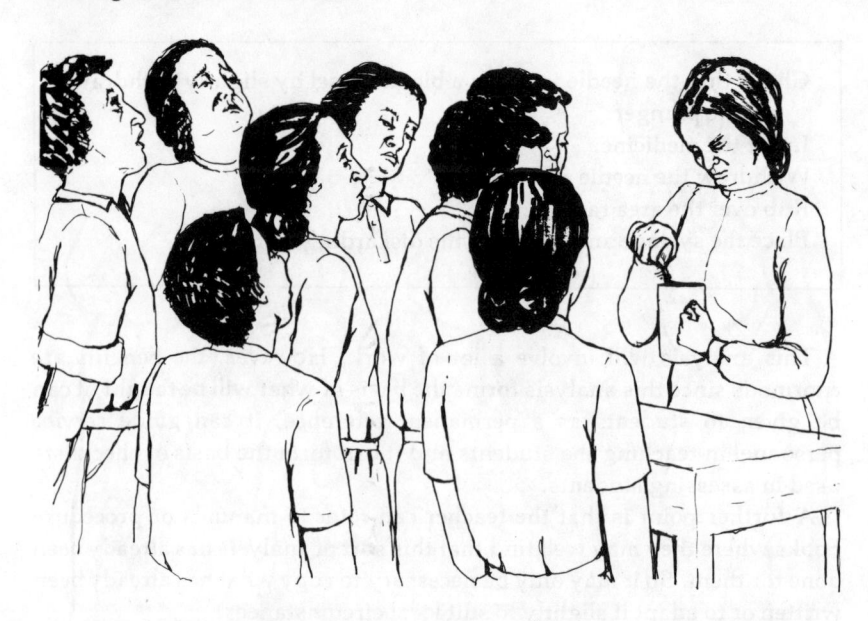

Figure 13.1 A demonstration should be visible to all students

skin and a real discarding tray. There is no reasonable excuse for not having any of the above. Whether a real patient is needed is a little bit different. Ideally a patient would be used, but in a classroom it might be sufficient to inject into a sponge or an orange. The teacher must certainly inject into something, to make absolutely clear what angle is used, how far the needle goes in, etc.

- A demonstration should proceed step-by-step. The steps must follow the task analysis precisely. The written list of sub-tasks should be available for the students to refer to during the demonstration.
- The teacher should describe what is being done and why. He should not need to explain some failure in the demonstration, such as, 'don't get this syringe unsterile, like I have, when you do this in the clinic', or, 'you really ought to wash your hands first, but as there's no water here I'm omitting this step'.

Demonstrating is a teacher-skill and like all skills it needs practice. Also, like all good lessons, it needs planning and preparation beforehand.

13.5 PROVIDING INITIAL EXPERIENCE IN EACH SKILL

After the initial demonstration and description of the manual skill, every student should perform the skill under close supervision.

This initial experience should be as soon as possible after the demonstration. Ideally it should take place in the same teaching session as the demonstration. This is because any delay between the demonstration and the students' first attempt at the task will make it more difficult for the students to remember what they should do.

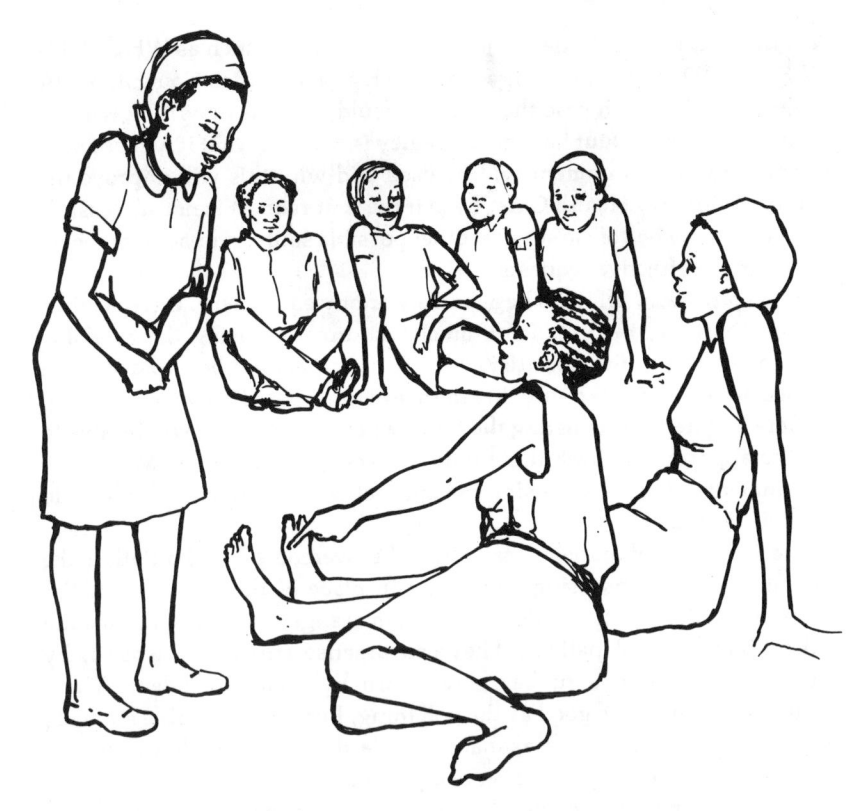

Figure 13.2 Students should initially practise under close supervision

During the initial experience the teacher should make sure that:

- all equipment, apparatus and patients are available for the students to perform the skill;
- there is sufficient time;
- detailed guidance and feedback is available to every student.

Each of these targets can be very difficult to achieve, so suggestions are given below.

(a) Providing Equipment, Apparatus and Patients—Simulation

Every manual skill in health care is carried out using equipment or is carried out on a patient. Therefore students cannot learn to perform manual skills unless they have the relevant equipment or a suitable patient.

This can seem impossible. A school may have just one or two microscopes for a class of thirty students or the training may take place an inconveniently long way away from patients.

The first thing to do is to try to obtain more sets of equipment. Sometimes old equipment is very rarely used and may be given to the training programme. Sometimes equipment can be borrowed from a health centre or a hospital. Sometimes money can be obtained to buy new equipment. This money should be requested from the Principal, the

Government, local charities, international agencies (such as WHO, UNICEF or UNDP) or national agencies (such as The British Council, SIDA or NORAD). In each case the request should be made in writing with an explanation given about how much money is needed, what it will be spent on and how the equipment will be used and why this will improve the quality of Primary Health Care. Even if the first request is not successful, the agency may be able to suggest other possible sources, or advise on how to write more effective requests.

If, despite every effort to beg, borrow or buy equipment, there is still a serious shortage, then students must take turns in using the available equipment. When this unsatisfactory situation cannot be avoided, then the teacher should make sure that the use of time is as efficient as possible. Prepare a roster or rota listing the times when each student will be able to use the apparatus. Check that students keep to these times. Make sure that students who are not using the apparatus have something else to do which is useful.

The shortage of patients can often be overcome by simulating the patients. This means using something in place of the real patient. For example, students can practise injecting an orange, a sponge or a cushion rather than the real patient. They can practise stitching a wound, by sewing up a cut in a rubber glove worn by another student. These simulations are not as good as the real thing, but they do enable students to learn the basic skill to a reasonable standard. In this way they are better prepared to go on and practise on real patients.

The other students in the class can also take the place of patients. Students can use other students when they first learn how to measure pulse and respiration rates, listen to heart sounds, examine conjunctiva, etc., etc.

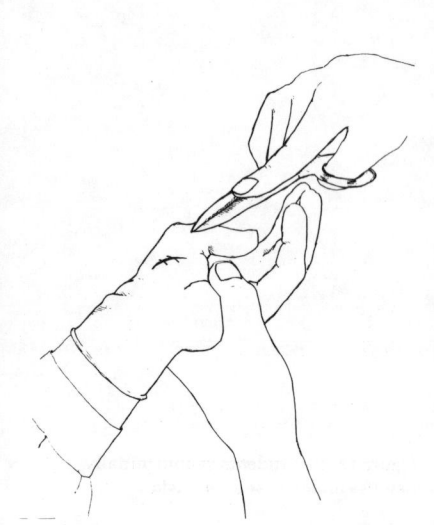

Figure 13.3 Simulation—students can practise stitching a wound by stitching a cut rubber glove

(b) Providing Enough Time

Learning manual skills (or other skills) takes longer than learning facts. So plenty of time is needed in the curriculum for this learning process. Often the curriculum does not allow sufficient time.

To overcome this problem, teachers can:

- Try to change the curriculum. Explain to the decision-makers why more time is needed. Explain that there is little point in having very detailed factual knowledge until students practise how to apply that knowledge in the practical situation. Ask for a larger proportion of time to practise skill, and less to learn facts.
- Try to minimise the waste of time which sometimes happens. This can happen when a lot of time is spent in travelling or when students have to wait for other students, teachers or health service staff to arrive.
- Encourage students to practise skills outside the timetabled hours. Students can often visit wards, casualty, out-patient departments or health centres during the evening, at weekends, at night or during vacations. They should be encouraged to do this.

- Start to teach manual skill from the beginning of the course—even the very first day. A student does not need to know the anatomy of the whole cardiovascular system before measuring a pulse rate. (In fact, the anatomy will make much more sense and will be learnt faster if the students already have some practical experience of pulses and listening to heart sounds.) So plan the order of the course to include as much learning of manual skills as possible in the early part of the course.

(c) Providing Detailed Guidance and Feedback—Practice in Pairs, Supervision

When students are learning how to perform manual skills it is essential to correct any faults in technique straight away. Students must not practise doing things in the wrong way.

Therefore detailed supervision is needed for every student and the supervisor should provide specific advice about what parts of the skill are being done well and also give advice about what is being done badly and how it can be done better.

The principle is simple—but how can it be put into practice? A teacher cannot provide detailed supervision for every student in a group of thirty or more.

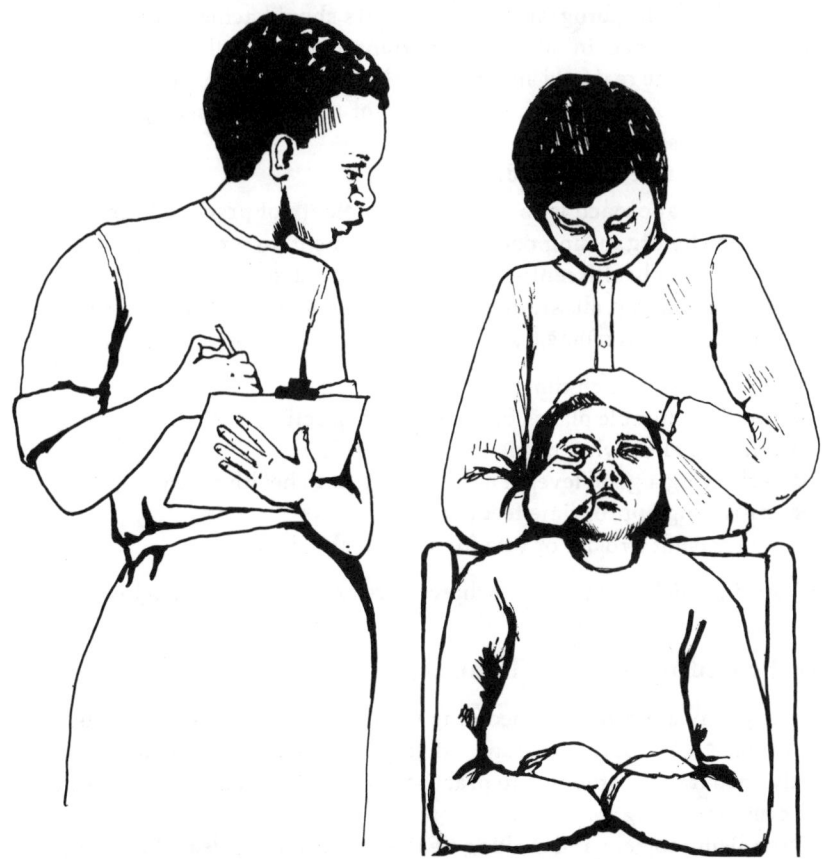

Figure 13.4 'Practise in pairs—one student examines the patient's conjunctiva whilst the second student observes using a checklist'

The teacher can arrange for practice in pairs. One student performs the skill whilst the other student observes and gives feedback. This feedback will be more helpful and accurate if a checklist based on a task analysis is provided.

The teacher can also arrange for more senior students or health service staff to help in supervising the students. Even though these people can be expected to have experience, an agreed checklist should still be provided. This will make the feedback more consistent and mean that everyone involved agrees on how the manual skill should be performed. (Such agreement is surprisingly rare even amongst experienced health workers.)

At the end of the initial experience stage, every student should have performed the skill. They should have reached a reasonable standard of competence—all major errors eliminated, but perhaps the students will be slow or a bit clumsy. They may only have practised the skill in a simulation and so have no experience with real patients.

At this stage the students are ready to learn how to increase the skill of their performance or to transfer to real patients. This stage is described below.

13.6 ARRANGING FOR FURTHER EXPERIENCE

During the training programme all students should achieve a high standard of competence in all the important manual skills. This means competence in the real field situation working under the normal conditions (the same equipment, the same amount of time and possibly the same amount of assistance).

This ideal is rarely achieved.

The overall approach is to give students plenty of practice in the field. This is done by organising periods of 'attachment' to service units such as wards, clinics or health centres. Even so, it is hard to achieve a high level of competence among all students for a variety of reasons. The major problems can be overcome by:

- providing enough time;
- finding suitable places for students to practise;
- making clear what needs to be practised;
- achieving a good level of co-operation with health service staff;
- providing appropriate feedback;
- organising a roster or rota for student attachments.

Ways in which these can be achieved are explained in turn below.

(a) Providing enough Time

This is partly a matter of scheduling within the curriculum (as discussed in section 13.5), partly making efficient use of the time available and partly encouraging students to practise skills during vacations, weekends and evenings or nights.

Organising rosters and making clear what needs to be learnt will help to achieve efficient use of time and these are discussed below.

(b) Finding Suitable Places for Students to Practise

This is often difficult. Teachers are often suspicious (sometimes rightly) of the quality of health care provided away from the teaching base. So they are reluctant to expose their students to the influence of health workers whose standards are not impeccable.

Yet some compromise is needed. Students must have experience in the field. So teachers should consider working with:

health centres and clinics;
specialist programmes (such as immunisation campaigns or malaria control programmes);
special diseases hospitals or clinics, such as leprosy, TB or infectious diseases clinics;
research organisations.

Some of these organisations may be independent of the government or voluntary and so there may be administrative difficulties—yet these difficulties are worth making every effort to overcome.

(c) Making Clear what Needs to be Learnt—Procedure Book, Checklists, Rating Scales

Unless students know what they should be practising, they are likely to spend a lot of time practising unnecessary skills, so it is essential to be very clear about what skills must be learnt.

Specifying what needs to be learnt involves producing a list of the skills. It also involves making clear what standard of performance is required.

The list of skills should be available as a result of the analysis described in section 13.3. The list can be rewritten and given to students in the form of a 'procedure book'.

The procedure book usually lists the skills to be practised, states what experience or practice is needed and may say where this practice can be obtained and also provides a space for a supervisor to sign when the practice has been completed.

Two extracts from a 'procedure book' are given overleaf.

The 'Procedure Book' should be supplemented by a checklist for each skill which explains the steps—and sometimes the standards—involved in each of the skills.

The checklists should be exactly the same as those used during the initial description of the skill. They can be referred to by the student to check his own performance. They can be used by other students or supervisors to help them give specific and consistent feedback.

It is suggested that appropriate checklists are developed locally in co-operation with health service staff. This will help to ensure that the training programme and the health service are working to the same standard and may help to develop greater co-operation between training and service staff.

The checklists—as mentioned before—should be based on a task analysis. However, it may help to reduce the work involved if checklists produced elsewhere are adapted (rather than starting from a blank sheet of paper). One source of checklists is available in *Assessing Health*

Workers' Performance by F. M. Katz and R. Snow (WHO Public Health Paper No. 72) published at Geneva in 1982.

An example of a checklist from this publication is given in table 13.1.

Two Examples from Procedure Books for Student Learners

I ... in the Ward

3.	Record the names of 10 patients on whom you have taken the T°, pulse and R.R.		Supervisor's signature
	1	2	
	3	4	
	5	6	Has done this
	7	8	....
	9	10	
4.	Record the names of 2 patients on whom you have dressed a wound		Has done this
	1	2	....
5.	Record the names of 3 patients on whom you have passed a naso-gastric tube		
	1	2	Has done this
	3		....

II ... in the Clinic

11.	Take the blood pressure of 10 antenatal patients (fill in the Card No. and results below)		Supervisor's signature
	1	2	
	3	4	
	5	6	Completed
	7	8	accurately
	9	10	....
12.	Time the foetal heart beat of 10 antenatal patients and record below		
	1	2	
	3	4	
	5	6	
	7	8	Correctly counted
	9	10	....

Note: In Frame I the supervisor is only asked to check whether a task has been done.

In Frame II the supervisor is asked to check whether it has been done competently.

Table 13.1

	Yes or Satisfactory	No or Unsatisfactory
Performance of safe, hygienic delivery		
1. Prepares for delivery		
• puts on clean apron		
• thoroughly scrubs hands		
• watches perineum for appearance of baby's head		
2. Prevents perineal laceration		
• applies gentle pressure to baby's head to slow the delivery		
• instructs mother to pant so as to reduce speed of delivery of head		
• applies gentle manual support to perineal area		
3. Delivers the baby		
• supports the head as it emerges		
• feels around baby's neck for cord		
• gently slips cord over head if it was found around neck		
• removes sac from head if it is present		
• wipes baby's eyes, nose and mouth with clean swab as soon as head emerges		
• supports baby as its body emerges		
• inverts baby to drain mucus		
• places baby on clean cloth cover between mother's legs		
4. Attends to umbilical cord		
• washes hands before manipulating cord		
• tests cord for cessation of pulsations		
• avoids contamination of cord ties		
• applies clean cord ties		
• ties square knots in applying cord ties		
• checks knots for security		
• lifts scissors by handles, avoiding contact with blades		
• cuts cord between the two cord ties		
• observes cord stump for bleeding		
• touches only edges of cord dressing		
• applies dressing with cord in 'turned up' position		
• avoids unsafe practices in cord care such as application of unclean materials, earth, saliva, ashes		
5. Prevents haemorrhage		
• puts baby to mother's breast to stimulate uterine contraction		
• identifies separation of placenta by watching for small gush of blood from birth canal		

(Continued overleaf)

Table 13.1 (contd)

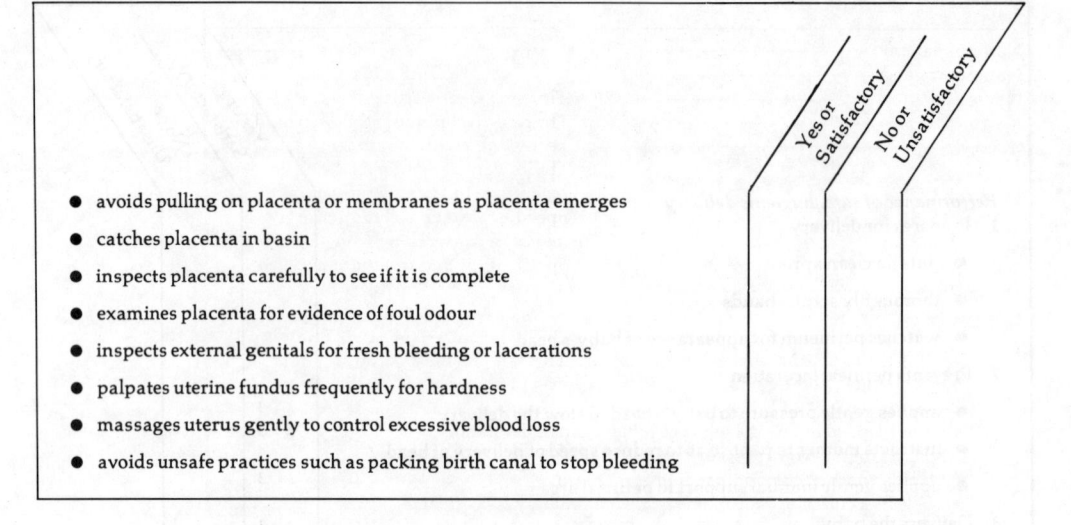

	Yes or Satisfactory	No or Unsatisfactory
avoids pulling on placenta or membranes as placenta emerges		
catches placenta in basin		
inspects placenta carefully to see if it is complete		
examines placenta for evidence of foul odour		
inspects external genitals for fresh bleeding or lacerations		
palpates uterine fundus frequently for hardness		
massages uterus gently to control excessive blood loss		
avoids unsafe practices such as packing birth canal to stop bleeding		

The above checklist is designed for a traditional birth attendant. It is part of a fuller checklist developed to assess the TBA's performance of a delivery in the home setting.

This checklist only records whether each stage was done or not done. 'Checklists' can be adapted to become 'Rating Scales' by putting in a rating of the quality of performing each stage.

Another example from the same publication is given in table 13.2 to illustrate a rating scale. Notice that the rating is made in general terms only here. It would be better (but much more difficult) to describe what 'adequate' means for each of the 14 'component tasks'.

(d) Achieving a Good Level of Co-operation with Health Services Staff

Health service staff are often busy and may regard students as a nuisance. They may feel that helping students to learn is not their job.

It is the job of the teacher to overcome all these possible antagonisms and win the co-operation of the health service staff.

This may be done by making personal visits and establishing a friendly relationship. The health service staff should be invited to join in planning the programme of student work in the field (and possibly they should be invited to comment on the whole training programme). This will help them to feel more involved. They will then be teaching on their own programme rather than somebody else's.

Students should realise that they also need to win the co-operation of the health service staff. So they should be as helpful as possible.

Health service staff will be an essential part of the supervision of students in most situations. So they should take part in designing

Table 13.2 Evaluation of blood pressure measurement for prenatal health care by maternal and child health trainee

Name of patient —————————— Date ——————
Name of trainee ——————————
Name of evaluator ————————————
Programme ————————————————
Site ——————————————————————

Rating scale
0 = This step was omitted
1 = The basic technique of this step needs to be reviewed with the student
2 = The student understands the basic technique, but needs more practice
3 = Speed, style, and technique are *adequate* for working with patients
4 = Speed, style, and technique excellent

I. *Direct observation*

Component tasks	Rating
1. Explains to the patient what will be done (e.g. 'This will feel tight on your arm, but it won't hurt'). Asks, 'Have you ever had your blood pressure taken?'	0 1 2 3 4
2. Explains blood pressure in language patient can understand.	0 1 2 3 4
3. Checks size of the blood pressure cuff.	
(a) Holds width of cuff against diameter of arm.	0 1 2 3 4
(b) Selects a cuff of appropriate size, approximately 20% greater than arm diameter.[1]	0 1 2 3 4
4. Rolls up sleeve of patient's garment so no material will be under cuff.	0 1 2 3 4
5. Centres cuff bladder over the brachial artery.	0 1 2 3 4
6. Positions and supports the arm at heart level.	
7. Takes a palpatory pulse.[2]	0 1 2 3 4
(a) Palpates radial or brachial artery.	0 1 2 3 4
(b) Inflates cuff until arterial pulse can no longer be felt.	0 1 2 3 4
(c) Inflates cuff 1.33 kPa (10 mmHg) higher.	0 1 2 3 4
(d) Deflates cuff at a rate no more than 0.4 kPa (3 mmHg) sec.	0 1 2 3 4
(e) Records kPa where arterial pulse is again palpated.	0 1 2 3 4
(f) Deflates cuff completely.	
8. Waits 30 seconds, allowing arm to rest (could take heart rate during this time).	0 1 2 3 4
9. Repositions arm at heart level.	0 1 2 3 4
10. Places diaphragm of stethoscope over brachial artery.	0 1 2 3 4
11. Inflates cuff to 2.67 kPa (20 mmHg) above palpatory pulse.	
12. Records auscultatory blood pressure.	0 1 2 3 4
(a) Records kPa where first sound heard.	0 1 2 3 4
(b) Records kPa where sounds muffle.	0 1 2 3 4
(c) Records kPa where sounds disappear.	0 1 2 3 4
13. Replaces arm at rest.	
14. Offers patient an opportunity to ask questions.	

II. *Auditory confirmation*

Student's reading ————————————————

Evaluator's reading ————————————————

Difference ——————————————————————

    Clinically significant   Y N ?

---
[1] If the cuff selected is too large, the blood pressure recorded will be erroneously low. If the cuff is too small, the reading will be erroneously high. Written short-answer or multiple-choice questions can be used to evaluate knowledge of this aspect.
[2] Used to obtain systolic estimate to avoid error from possible auscultatory gap.

checklists or rating scales. They should meet with the teachers to agree on standards of performance. Overall, the distinction between teachers and service staff should be minimised as far as possible.

(e) Providing Appropriate Feedback

This is the key to rapid learning of manual skills. The feedback should be specific (i.e. detailed and precise) and should be offered as a way of helping to improve performance—not as a means of finding fault. The feedback should also be based on a high standard of performance.

The tools to use in giving feedback are the checklists and rating scales described above.

The people who should use the tools are:

- the learner himself;
- other students;
- health service staff who supervise the students;
- occasionally the teacher.

(f) Organising a Roster or Rota for Student Attachments

This is a way of making sure that each student gets a variety of experience. It also makes sure that each host or health service department only has a small number of students to supervise.

A simple roster is given in table 13.3. Each of the 24 students is identified by a number 1 to 24. There are 8 places for students to work in and they will go to each place for 2 days in each of the 8 weeks.

Table 13.3

	MCH Clinic in Health Centre X	MCH Clinic in Health Centre Y	Home visits with Public Health Nurse X	Home visits with PHN Y	Home visits with PHN Z	Mobile Immunisation Team	Medical Records Unit in Health Centre X	Maternity Unit in Health Centre X
Week 1	A	B	C	D	E	F	G	H
Week 2	B	C	D	E	F	G	H	A
Week 3	C	D	E	F	G	H	A	B
Week 4	D	E	F	G	H	A	B	C
Week 5	E	F	G	H	A	B	C	D
Week 6	F	G	H	A	B	C	D	E
Week 7	G	H	A	B	C	D	E	F
Week 8	H	A	B	C	D	E	F	G

Group A is students 1, 2 and 3, Group B is students 4, 5 and 6, etc.

The teacher should prepare rosters like the example above.

They should then visit each of the locations whilst the students are there. This will help the teacher to check that the roster is working. It will give the teacher a chance to talk with the health service personnel, to develop co-operation and to check that there are no organisational problems. The teacher will also be able to make sure that the standards being applied in the checklists are at about the right level.

Naturally the health service staff must be willing to accept the students and to supervise them properly. Teachers must make sure well in advance that they can rely on this co-operation.

13.7 ASSESSING WHETHER STUDENTS HAVE LEARNT THE MANUAL SKILLS

Throughout the teaching of manual skills, the importance of assessing students' performances in order to give feedback has been stressed. So assessment and teaching cannot be regarded as separate. Good teaching depends on making helpful assessments.

The basic technique of assessing manual skills can only be to observe the student performing the skill and make a judgement about the quality of the performance. Asking the student to describe or write down how he would do something is virtually a waste of time.

The problems in assessment of manual skills do not therefore concern the basic technique (observation). The problems are only to do with how to make the observation more reliable and how to overcome the very real practical difficulties of organising and making enough time available.

There is one additional point. Manual skills are often performed by health workers as part of a more complex task. For example, weighing a baby involves manual skills in handling the baby and setting up the weighing scale. But the whole skill will also involve communication with the mother and decision making about the implications of the child's weight. Because the real tasks in the field involve a variety of skills it is quite appropriate to assess the student's ability to perform the complete task rather than separate the manualskill part from the communication part.

Increasing the reliability of assessment depends on achieving a uniform standard amongst the different observers/examiners. Studies have shown that this is very difficult to achieve and that in fact the score awarded to a student can vary widely from one examiner to another.

The main way in which this situation can be improved is to use checklists or rating scales. Examples of these were given earlier in this chapter. These instruments are not magical. They will only work if the people using them are taught how to use them and are willing to use them.

Therefore it is important to have meetings to discuss the use of checklists/rating scales and to agree on what standards are required to reach 'satisfactory' for each of the items on the checklist.

Effective checklists or rating scales will usually not contain more than 20 items—and checklists or rating scales can be as short as 5 or 6 items. The length has to be limited because the observer cannot record more than this number of items. (This restriction does not apply if the task takes a long time to perform and is always performed in the same order.)

Effective checklists and rating scales have usually been developed by several people who have adapted and improved the original version. So do make checklists available for comment and revision.

Scoring the student's performance should come *after* the initial recording of what happened. The simple way to score checklists is to give 1 mark for each item carried out satisfactorily. So in the performance of a 'safe hygienic delivery' there are 36 items. If the student does 25 of these items then the student's score is 25 out of 36.

Should this student pass?

In many exams the pass mark is 50% or 60%, corresponding to 18/36 or 22/36. So maybe the student should pass.

Well, this is plainly ridiculous and illustrates how meaningless the usual 50% or 60% pass mark really is. If 50% was the pass, a student might be qualified, yet not have done anything about the umbilical cord at all.

So if the simple system of 1 point for every item is used, then the pass mark must be much higher than 60%—possibly as high as 90% or even 95%. To set the pass mark, the teacher should decide what is an adequate, safe performance; what things could be left out without causing too much danger. For example, 'catches placenta in basin' is clearly desirable—but would it cause serious risk if it was not done? On the other hand 'avoids unsafe practices in cord care such as application of unclean materials, earth, saliva, ashes', is clearly of great importance. By considering what is safe and important, a rational pass mark can be obtained. Note that the pass mark might be different from checklist to checklist.

Another technique is to categorise each item as 'essential', 'important' and 'desirable'. Then the student will only pass if every essential item is performed successfully and, say, 80% of the important items plus, say, 50% of the desirable items. This is probably the ideal, but it is fairly complicated to administer.

Other variations can give 3 points to every essential item, 2 to the important and 1 to the desirable items.

Similar approaches to scoring rating scales apply. Where the rating is on a 5, 4, 3, 2, 1, 0 basis, the scores for each item can simply be added together.

The scoring can be made more appropriate—but more complicated—by doubling the rating on some items (so it becomes a 10, 8, 6, 4, 2, 0 scale). This gives more weight to items which the examiner feels are more important.

The pass mark for a rating scale assessment may be in the region of 60%, although higher standards should not be rejected on grounds of tradition or precedent. Again the principle is to think how many points a barely satisfactory health worker would obtain. If this person would get 70% on that rating scale, then 70% should be the pass mark.

Making time for assessment is crucial, yet often not easy to achieve. For example, suppose there are 20 manual skills to be learned and 30 students. If a single teacher observed each student doing each manual skill he would need 600 observations.

Since the average time taken for a manual skill might be 10 min, 600 observations would take 6000 min or 100 h!! This means that it would take a teacher two weeks of full time work (50 h a week) to assess the competence of 30 students.

Courses and teachers do not have that much time to spare.
How can this difficulty be overcome?

Continuous Assessment

Teachers should assess manual skills throughout the course. Assessment of manual skills cannot be done adequately if it is only done during a practical examination at the end of term or the end of the course.

Assessment of manual skills should take place all through the course.

Using a 'Procedure Book' (see sub-section 13.6c)

Each student is given a list of manual skills or a procedure book, and is told to gain as much practice as he can find.

As he feels himself to be competent in each skill he approaches the teachers or health staff member and asks for an assessment. When he is found competent a mark is scored on his list (or in his book).

By the end of the course the student will have acquired competence in all the skills on the list. And this will be an essential part of the final assessment for qualification.

Assessment by Working Staff

The PHC teacher can ask the health centre, hospital or clinic staff to help him in assessing the skills of his students. This is especially useful when those staff are also involved in the training of the students in manual skills. This is because assessing the students will encourage the staff to train the students well.

The staff should be given copies of:
(1) the students' procedure list;
(2) the assessment checklists/rating scales.

They should also meet with the teachers to discuss standards of competence required.

Using an Objective Structured Practical Examination (OSPE)

The OSPE is a way of organising assessment of all practical skills in an intensive way. During one morning or afternoon a wide range of skills can be assessed for every student in quite a large group.

The technique is described in detail in chapter 8. The only points to emphasise here are:

- The technique is equally appropriate for manual skills as for communication skills and decision-making skills.
- The technique can be used during the learning process, possibly at the end of one part of the course. It can also be used in the final assessment of students.

SUMMARY

- Manual skills are crucially important in health care.
- The main principle of teaching manual skills is to provide a lot of practice for students.
- This practice should be observed. Students, health service staff and teachers can co-operate in observing. The quality of the feedback given to learners is critically important and can be improved by using checklists and rating scales.
- Assessment of students must be based on observation of students performing the skills.

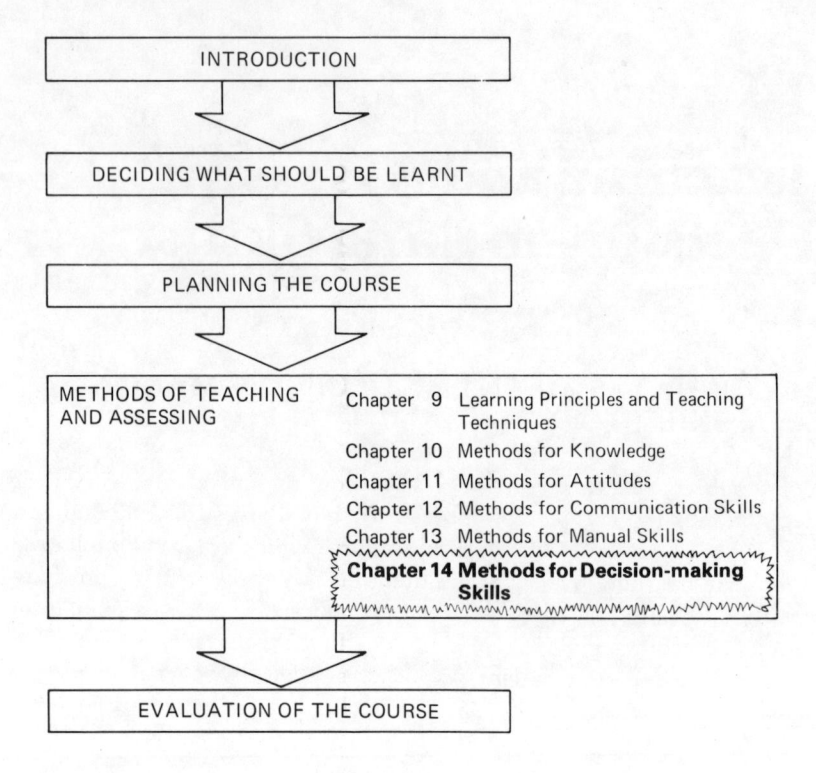

```
┌─────────────────────────┐
│      INTRODUCTION       │
└─────────────────────────┘
             ↓
┌─────────────────────────┐
│ DECIDING WHAT SHOULD BE LEARNT │
└─────────────────────────┘
             ↓
┌─────────────────────────┐
│    PLANNING THE COURSE  │
└─────────────────────────┘
             ↓
┌──────────────────────────────────────────────────────────┐
│ METHODS OF TEACHING    Chapter  9  Learning Principles and Teaching
│ AND ASSESSING                      Techniques
│                        Chapter 10  Methods for Knowledge
│                        Chapter 11  Methods for Attitudes
│                        Chapter 12  Methods for Communication Skills
│                        Chapter 13  Methods for Manual Skills
│                        **Chapter 14 Methods for Decision-making**
│                                    **Skills**
└──────────────────────────────────────────────────────────┘
             ↓
┌─────────────────────────┐
│  EVALUATION OF THE COURSE │
└─────────────────────────┘
```

CONTENTS

14.1	What is Meant by Decision-making Skills?	199
14.2	What are the Skills of Decision Making?	201
14.3	General Methods of Teaching Decision-making Skills	202
14.4	Analysing the Decision-making Skills	202
14.5	Describing and Demonstrating the Skills to the Learner	203
14.6	Providing Practice in Decision Making	203
14.7	Brain-storming	205
14.8	Snowballing	207
14.9	Case Histories, Case Studies and Patient-management Problems	209
14.10	Flowcharts	211
14.11	Games and Simulations	212
14.12	Role-play Exercises	213
14.13	Observed Field Work	213
14.14	Field Work with a Supervisor	214
14.15	Assessing Decision-making Skills	214

14
Teaching and Assessing Decision-making Skills

14.1 WHAT IS MEANT BY DECISION-MAKING SKILLS?

Some aspects of health care are rather routine and involve very little decision making. For example, measuring blood pressure or administering a vaccine are fairly standard procedures which are usually followed through in the same sequence time after time. But these are fairly unusual. Nearly all health care involves decision making. Even these examples of routine procedures require health workers to make decisions from time to time. Suppose that the patient's blood pressure is high. What should the health worker do? Should the patient be told, and if so, how much should be said?

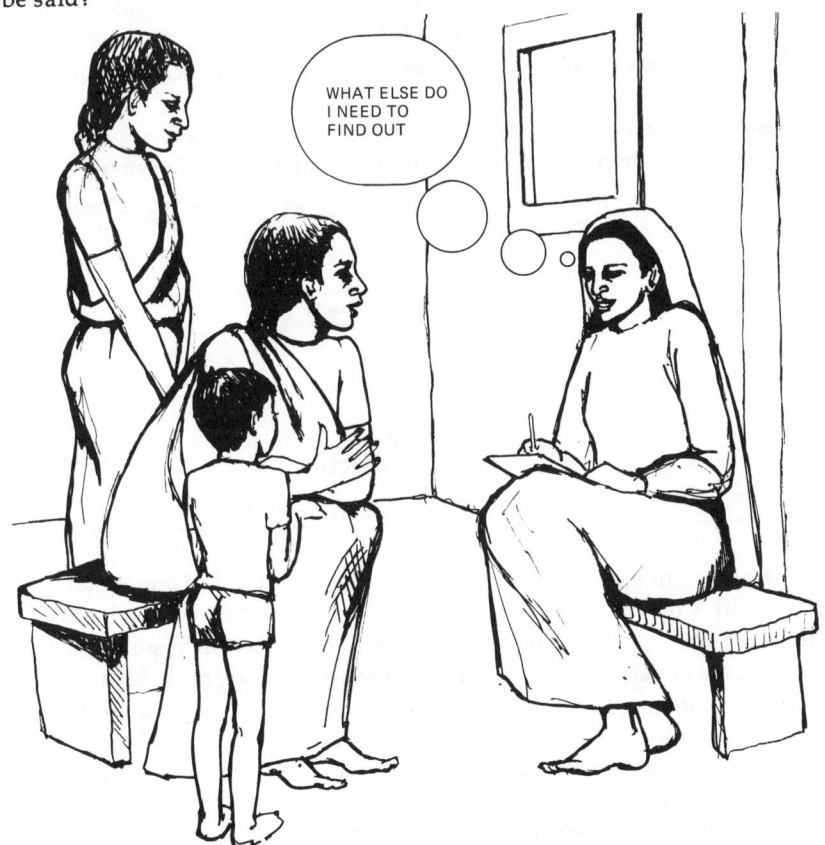

Figure 14.1 Health workers are making decisions whilst they take a history

Other examples of health care work involve decision making much more obviously. All diagnosis and individual patient management clearly involves the health worker in frequent decision making. Suppose a patient comes to a health centre and says to the medical assistant, 'I have a headache'. At this point the medical assistant must decide what question to ask next. Then, in due course, a decision must be taken about the probable cause of the headache and what should be done about it.

Other types of health care work also involve making decisions. Where is the best site in a village for a well? What food could this family afford to buy? What drugs need to be ordered? Is this child really malnourished? Should this pregnant woman be referred for more specialised treatment? How can this shopkeeper be persuaded to keep his shop in a cleaner condition? Who would be the best person to advise this farmer about storing his crops?

In all these cases the health worker will need to take into account some factual knowledge, e.g. in the case of siting a well this will include knowledge of geological features which determine where water is likely to be found, knowledge of criteria for siting wells away from latrines or other sewage disposal sites, knowledge of criteria to apply such as convenience of village people, etc.

The factual knowledge must then be applied to the specific situation. In this case the geological features must be recognised and interpreted, the sites of latrines and sewage disposal should be recorded and villagers' requirements for convenience identified.

Then all these different factors must be taken into account and a site selected.

This whole process of remembering facts or knowledge, applying it to the specific situation and coming to a decision is the decision-making process.

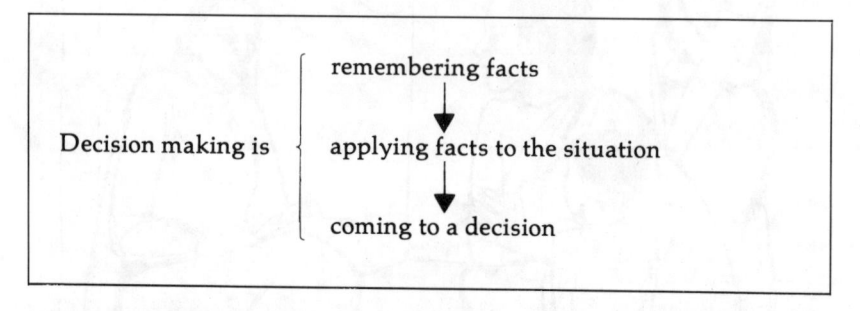

Decision making is
- remembering facts
↓
- applying facts to the situation
↓
- coming to a decision

Some health authorities try to reduce the need for decision making by the health workers. They do this by specifying procedures which must be followed and by providing manuals or flowcharts which guide history taking, examination and diagnosis. These attempts are probably useful as they make it more likely that the more common and more serious mistakes will be avoided. But even so, health workers will be left with many decisions to make every day, and so decision-making skill is important. Moreover it must be learnt.

To make good decisions one needs both the relevant knowledge and also the skill to use that knowledge in reaching the decision.

14.2 WHAT ARE THE SKILLS OF DECISION MAKING?

How do people make decisions? This may seem a very simple question, answered by saying, 'They think about the problem and reach a conclusion'.

But what does 'thinking about a problem' mean? Can the ability to 'think' be taught?

These are very profound questions and the full answers are not known. However, some incomplete answers can be given—and although they are not complete they are enough to guide teaching of decision-making skills.

There are some strategies that everyone can use in decision-making. These include:

- identifying relevant information;
- distinguishing between facts and opinions;
- listing advantages and disadvantages;
- predicting consequences of a solution or course of action;
- recognising patterns (e.g. a pattern of symptoms may be recognised as being typical of a specific disease);
- following an algorithm or flowchart.

(This means following a set of rules which guide decision making.)

For example, an algorithm for diagnosing the cause of a cough in children is given below.

> 'If the cough is of less than 4 weeks duration and there is dyspnoea with either creps or fever then the most likely cause is pneumonia. If there is no dyspnoea but the child wheezes then the diagnosis is bronchitis or asthma . . .'

(Part of an algorithm for diagnosing the cause of a cough.)
The description can be written more usefully as a flowchart.

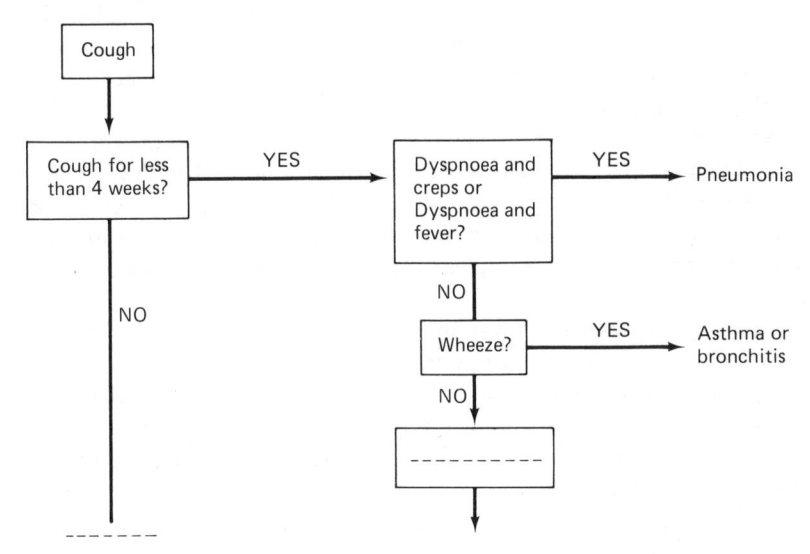

(Part of a flowchart adapted from *Diagnostic Pathways in Clinical Medicine—An Epidemiological Approach to Clinical Problems*, B. J. Essex, Churchill Livingstone, 1977.)

This is a very brief and greatly simplified list of some decision-making strategies yet it is already enough to suggest some ways of teaching decision-making skills. For example, the first strategy (i.e. 'identifying relevant information'), can be helped by telling students that they are responsible for reducing the incidence of malaria or some other relevant disease in the district round the school. Then ask them to write down as many relevant facts about malaria and about the district as they can. This exercise will tend to expand the students' ability to take into account a wider range of information when reaching decisions.

For more detailed information on decision making the reader might like to read *Teaching Thinking* by Edward de Bono, published by Penguin Books (1978).

14.3 GENERAL METHODS OF TEACHING DECISION-MAKING SKILLS

The pattern for teaching decision-making skills is rather similar to the pattern for communication skills. This involves:

(1) analysing the decision-making skills;
(ii) describing and demonstrating the skills to the learner;
(iii) providing practice in decision-making skills and providing feedback on the skill;
(iv) assessing whether the students have achieved sufficient competence.

14.4 ANALYSING THE DECISION-MAKING SKILLS

As for each of the other types of skill, the teacher should analyse exactly what is involved in decision making. This is rather idealistic and impractical since teachers may well have experience in analysing manual skills such as giving an injection, but they are much less likely to have analysed the process of reaching decisions. So in practice what can teachers do when they prepare to teach decision-making skills?

The starting point is to think about the situations in which the students will need to make decisions when they are fully trained as health workers. (This can be distracting because the natural tendency is to then think about *what* the student will need to know—rather than *how* the student will *use* what he knows.) Examples of these situations are given in section 14.1.

Then think through the ways in which a health worker reaches the decision. Do any of the strategies given in section 14.2 seem relevant?

In this way teachers can build up a picture of the situation where decisions need to be made and of the way in which the decisions can be made. This picture can now be used as a basis for developing teaching/learning exercises.

14.5 DESCRIBING AND DEMONSTRATING THE SKILLS TO THE LEARNER

The teacher can use one or two of the situations identified in his analysis of decision-making skills (as in section 14.4). This situation can be used as a case study in the following way.

> 'The people living in Village X have contacted you and asked for your advice about where they should dig a well. Make a list of the information you know about siting wells. Make another list of the information you would want to find out about in the village.'

This exercise would allow the teacher to illustrate the skills of gathering a wide range of information and of selecting that information which is relevant.

> The teacher could then draw a detailed map of the village and mark on it a proposed site for the well. The teacher could then ask 'Make a list of the advantages and disadvantages of siting the well in this place'.

This exercise could be used by the teacher to illustrate the skills of predicting consequences and thinking through advantages and disadvantages from different points of view.

The essential point is that at some time in the course students should be told explicitly what decision-making skills and strategies they can use. This is especially important if the students' previous learning has been in schools where the emphasis has been mainly on remembering facts, rather than applying their knowledge.

14.6 PROVIDING PRACTICE IN DECISION MAKING

It is certainly difficult for teachers to describe decision-making skills or to demonstrate them, since these skills are to some extent sub-conscious and imprecise. Therefore this inevitable weakness should be compensated for, by providing frequent opportunities for practising the skills of decision-making.

This can be achieved partly by using a certain style of teaching throughout all the teaching sessions and partly by arranging specific exercises and experiences.

The style which should be adopted throughout teaching is to repeatedly ask students questions which require them to apply knowledge and reach decisions. When teachers ask these questions they should aim to make sure that all students answer each question. Compare the teacher who says, 'Can anyone tell me . . .?' with the teacher who says, 'Please write down on a scrap of paper . . .'. In the first case a few bright and eager students will have an answer—but only one student's answer will be

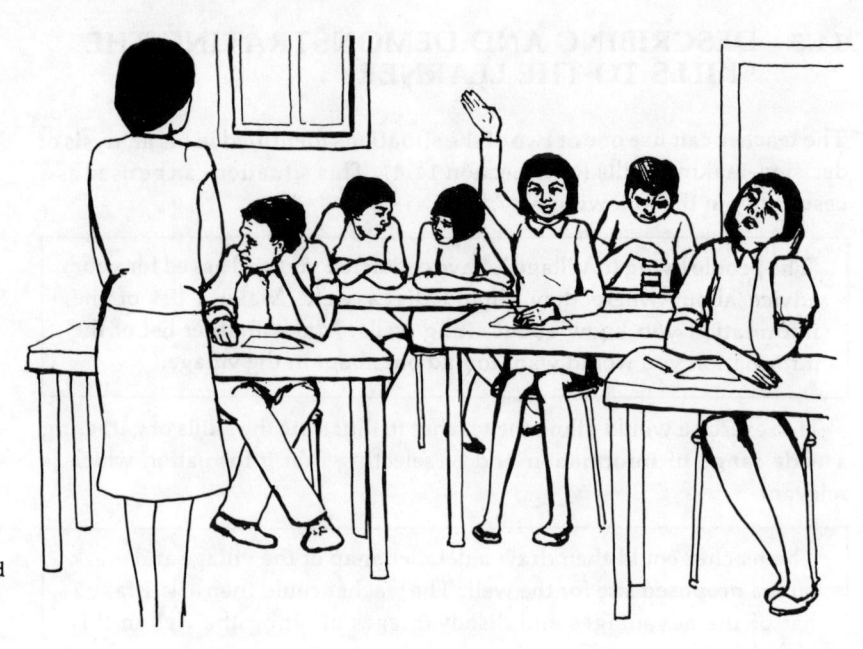

Figure 14.2 When a question is asked to the class as a whole, only one student gives the answer . . .

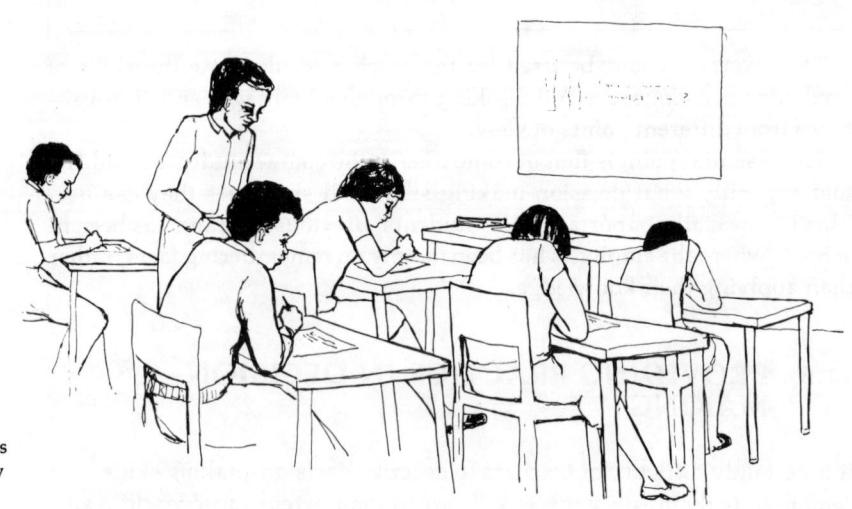

Figure 14.3 . . . but if every student is asked to write down the answer, every student has to reach a decision

given. In the second case the teacher can walk round and have a look at several different answers. All—or at least most—of the students will actually commit themselves to an answer.

This style of teaching provides continuing practice in reaching decisions throughout a course.

There are also techniques for providing practice in decision-making skills which can be used as the main content of a teaching session. These include:

Brain-storming (section 14.7)
Snowballing (section 14.8)
Case histories, case studies, and patient-management problems (section 14.9)

Flowcharts (section 14.10)
Games and simulation exercises (section 14.11)
Role-play exercises (section 14.12)
Observed field work (section 14.13)
Field work with a supervisor (section 14.14)

These specific techniques are in an order which reflects the increasing reality in the situation (i.e. the exercises become closer and closer to the real work environment) and an increasing degree of responsibility for the student. This second aspect is important as there is all the difference in the world between on the one hand making decisions in a paper and pencil exercise about what you would do if a patient was brought to a health centre unconscious with serious facial injuries after a road traffic accident and on the other hand actually making these decisions in the real situation. Training should prepare the students to make decisions in the real world.

14.7 BRAIN-STORMING

Brain-storming is the name sometimes given to general discussion sessions during which people express ideas freely. This is a pity because true brain-storming is a much more precise technique that has powerful advantages.

A true brain-storm is a technique for generating ideas or a variety of solutions to a problem. It has a place in decision making as it helps to increase the range of factors taken into account in reaching a decision.

It is best used with groups of between 5 and 20 students.

There are four distinct stages in the brain-storm which must be followed in order.

The Stages in a Brain-storm

Stage 1: Defining the Problem for which Solutions are Required

All members of the brain-storm group must be clear about the kinds of ideas that they are trying to produce. Examples of problems might be:

What factors should be considered when deciding whether to refer a pregnant woman for a hospital delivery?
OR
What might persuade a mother to breast feed her baby
OR
What are the advantages (or the disadvantages) of a piped water supply in a village?

(Continued overleaf)

> ### Stage 2: The Brain-storm itself
>
> The teacher or group leader (who may be a student) invites suggestions or ideas.
> He records these on a board or an overhead projector as quickly as possible.
> All ideas are recorded whoever makes them and however silly or inappropriate they may seem. The ideas should be recorded even if they have been suggested previously.
>
> *No discussion or clarification of any kind is permitted*
>
> This stage continues until the ideas are exhausted.
> The Chairman should have some ideas to suggest when the flow of ideas from the members slows down. This is done to start the flow again.
>
> ### Stage 3: Review
>
> Each of the suggestions is reviewed so that:
>
> (1) It is clear to everyone what the suggestion is (sometimes only a word will be recorded to represent a complex idea).
> (2) A decision is made to keep the suggestion on the list for future discussion, or to throw it out. The aim is not to decide whether the idea is good or not, simply to decide whether it is worth discussing. Repetition of ideas is one reason for throwing out suggestions.
>
> ### Stage 4: Discussion
>
> The remaining ideas are discussed to decide which suggestions to accept and to develop the ideas further.

In the examples above the brain-storm should yield a lot of suggestions and probably rather more suggestions than any one of the students could have provided. This process therefore is a way of enlarging the students' view of what is involved and is likely to help them to consider more factors in future decision making.

Why does brain-storming work?

The central brain-storm works because many people are either consciously or sub-consciously afraid of putting forward ideas in case they are ridiculed or the ideas are just not good enough. In the brain-storm all ideas are accepted and the natural tendency to evaluate an idea before expressing it is 'switched off'. In this way the participants become less inhibited.

Further, the speed at which the ideas are produced itself stimulates more ideas. Someone has a foolish idea, but someone else builds on that idea to produce something better.

Here are some suggestions for other brain-storming sessions.

- How can you help people to remember the correct quantities of sugar, salt and water in Oral Rehydration Solutions?
- What would you want to find out from a patient who complained of headache? (or any other common or general complaint such as tiredness, fever, cough).
- What could community health workers do to increase the proportion of children who are immunised in their community?

14.8 SNOWBALLING

'Snowballing' is another group activity which can develop some of the skills of decision making such as identifying advantages and disadvantages or predicting consequences. It is best used with groups of between 8 and 32 people.

It is called snowballing because it is rather like when a snowball rolls down a hill. As it rolls it gathers more snow and gets larger and larger (so it is not a very helpful name for people living in tropical countries!). In the same way, the snowball technique starts with very small groups of people which join together and get larger and larger.

Stages in Snowballing

Stage 1

Start with a clear statement of the situation and what everybody has to do. This might be, 'Think about the district of X (at this point, the teacher should display a map of this district and give some background data about patterns of disease, etc.). In X there is some money available which can be spent on immunisation campaigns
OR
health education
OR
an extension to the District Hospital.
There isn't enough money to make it worth while sharing it between these projects. Think what the advantages and disadvantages would be for each course of action'.
Or a rather simpler situation:
'Part of your job is to survey the health hazards in the community. But there never seems to be time to do this because there are so many people coming to the clinic. Think what might happen if the clinic was closed for 2 afternoons every week in order to do the survey.'

(Continued overleaf)

Stage 2

A few minutes (5–10) is allowed for everybody individually to think of advantages and disadvantages or to think of what might happen. The students can be shown as separate circles:

O O O O O O O O O O O O O O

Stage 3

The individuals form groups of 2 and combine their ideas. They should identify where they have essentially the same idea, where there are new ideas and possibly where some ideas should be rejected. It is useful to ask the students to produce a written agreed list.

OO   OO   OO   OO   OO   OO   OO

(Each O represents one student. So here students are in groups of 2)

Stage 4

The pairs can now join to form fours. The teacher may change the task slightly at this stage and ask the group of four to reach a decision about what thewould do (i.e. decide which activity to spend the money on, or whether to close the clinic).

Because there were 14 students to start with in this example, there will now have to be two groups of only 3.

OOOO   OOO   OOO   OOOO

Stage 5

As a final exercise one of the groups of 4 should try to persuade the members of another group of 4 or 3 why their decision is right.

OOOOOOO OOOOOOO

The conclusion is for the teacher to review the discussion and try to draw out:
(1) The range of advantages or reasons offered by the students.
(2) The pattern of arguments used to justify the decision.

Used in this way snowballing gives every student practice in thinking about what factors to consider, using these factors in reaching a decision and listening to the arguments of other people. These learning objectives should be explained to the students—possibly at the end of the exercise—so that they will realise how the snowballing can help them in their own decision making in the field.

The teacher's role in the snowball is:

- to identify the situation for discussion;
- to keep time and control of the students so that they form new groups quickly;

- to listen to discussions in some of the groups to prepare for the final review;
- to review the conclusions and the arguments used.

14.9 CASE HISTORIES, CASE STUDIES AND PATIENT-MANAGEMENT PROBLEMS

Case histories and case studies are esentially the same thing, the only difference being that case histories usually refer to patients and case studies to situations.

Case studies are basically a description of what happened in a specific situation (e.g. how a specific malaria control programme was planned and implemented. What the results of the programme were). Similarly a case history is a description of a specific patient (presenting symptoms, history of the complaint, social history, preliminary diagnosis, examinations and tests performed, treatment provided, outcome). In this form, case studies and case histories can provide useful examples to illustrate general principles.

When they are used to help teach decision making, the full case history or case study is interrupted at a particular point and students (either individually or in groups) are asked, 'What would you do now?' or, 'What factors so far provided will be relevant to your decision about what to do?'

(Note that the Brain-storming and Snowballing exercises started off with brief case studies or case histories.)

One way of using case studies is to provide the initial information, then ask a question. The question is answered by individual students or by groups of students. Then some more of the case study is provided and a second question asked.

An example is given below.

A Case Study

Mrs A brought her 15-month-old son to the Health Centre clinic. She said that her son had been suffering from diarrhoea for a period of 5 days and that her son now seemed weak, tired and listless.

Question 1. What condition should you suspect at this point?

(Several reasonable answers could be given here, but probably the most important condition to worry about is dehydration.)

The case history now continues . . .
Dehydration was considered at this point.

Question 2. What would you look for to decide whether the child was dehydrated?

(After checking that all major signs and symptoms have been given, the case history continues.)

(Continued overleaf)

> The child was found to be dehydrated and it was decided that it would be possible to treat the dehydration with oral rehydration therapy in the health centre. Mrs A was asked to help in providing this therapy.
>
> Question 3. What are the advantages of treating dehydration in the Health Centre, rather than referring to a hospital?
>
> ———
>
> Question 4. What key things would you like Mrs A to learn whilst she is helping to treat her son?
>
> ———
>
> (The case history can continue as long as is necessary to cover the main points of the teaching session.)

When case studies or case histories are organised in this way, with several stages and a question after each stage, they are often called Patient Management Problems.

The main point of providing case histories is to show how the facts or knowledge learnt during the course can be applied in the field situation.

The role of the teacher is to bring out some of the decision-making strategies which the health workers can use and show how these apply. This is much more important than teaching the answers to the problems. So in this case, the teacher can use Question 1 to help them think about a wide range of conditions related to the diarrhoea and to help them think about other information they might collect. Question 3 directly asks them to list advantages and disadvantages, so the teacher should ensure that a wide range of factors is given (i.e. consider the mother's and the child's point of view, consider the practical and cost factors as well as the purely medical issues).

Case histories and case studies are usually most successful when they are based on real cases which the teacher (or perhaps one of the students) has actually dealt with. This makes sure that the cases are realistic and that it is possible to provide additional background details.

Case studies and case histories can be presented in a written form as a separate handout. Another way is to write the information on an overhead projector transparency (a big advantage here is that it becomes easy to show just one stage at a time). Another way is simply to read the case history. This is not very satisfactory unless it is supplemented by key points written on the board. For all these presentation methods it is desirable—but rather time-consuming—to bring the case histories to life by showing 35 mm slides of the situation or possibly playing a tape recording of the conversation. Naturally, where it is feasible, the actual patient should be in the teaching session with the students.

When case histories are used to teach decision making the crucial point is that the teachers must always be asking the students to think, to answer questions, to suggest possible solutions. It is almost a waste of time for the teacher to say, 'This is Mr A. He is 35 years old. He complained of . . . I diagnosed . . . and treated him with . . .' Instead the teacher must invite all the students to suggest what information to obtain in the history taking, to suggest what tests are needed, to put forward diagnoses.

14.10 FLOWCHARTS

Flowcharts are charts which are designed to help health workers reach a decision about treatment or diagnosis.

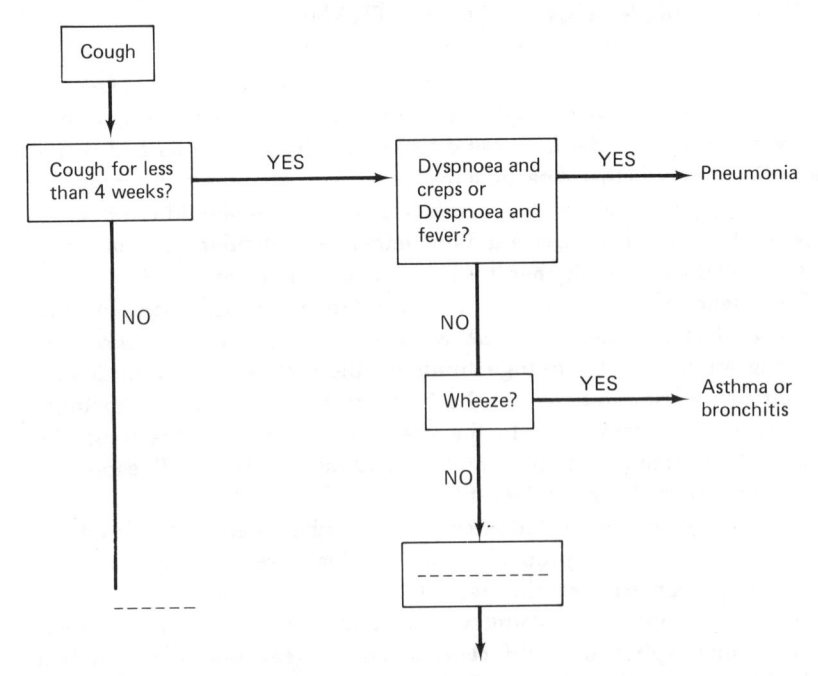

```
          ┌────────┐
          │ Cough  │
          └───┬────┘
              ▼
     ┌─────────────┐   YES    ┌──────────────┐   YES
     │ Cough for   │─────────▶│ Dyspnoea and │─────────▶ Pneumonia
     │ less than   │          │ creps or     │
     │ 4 weeks?    │          │ Dyspnoea and │
     └──────┬──────┘          │ fever?       │
            │                 └──────┬───────┘
            │ NO                     │ NO
            │                        ▼
            │                 ┌──────────┐  YES
            │                 │ Wheeze?  │─────────▶ Asthma or bronchitis
            │                 └────┬─────┘
            │                      │ NO
            │                      ▼
            │                 ┌ ─ ─ ─ ─ ┐
            │                 │         │
            │                 └ ─ ─ ─ ─ ┘
            ▼                      ▼
```

(Part of a flowchart adapted from *'Diagnostic Pathways in Clinical Medicine—An Epidemiological Approach to Clinical Problems'*, B. J. Essex, Churchill Livingstone, 1977)

This chart guides a health worker about the questions and examinations when a patient complains of a cough. In this chart, the first question to ask is 'How long have you had the cough?' (Note this is not specifically shown on the chart, but it is implied.) If the patient tells the health worker that he has only been coughing for five days, then the health worker knows that the cough is for less than 4 weeks and so goes on to find out about dyspnoea, creps and fever. If the patient has dyspnoea *and* creps or if the patient has dyspnoea *and* fever, then the health worker would diagnose pneumonia. If not, the health worker goes on to find out about wheezing.

The value of flowcharts in teaching and their value in the field as an aid to diagnosis are both controversial. Experiments in the field seem to show that flowcharts can increase both the accuracy and speed of diagnosis. Yet in a number of situations they are unpopular both with patients and with health workers. This may be because they are unfamiliar and it will take time for people to get used to using flowcharts.

In teaching, the value of flowcharts needs to be explored in more detail. At this time, it seems likely that teaching students how to use flowcharts is desirable. This will give the students an extra tool to help them in their health care work. (It does seem as though health workers who are not taught how to use flowcharts in their initial training, will be unlikely to start using them later.) It could also be argued that using flowcharts during the training period will help students to be more logical and systematic in their thinking and decision making.

14.11 GAMES AND SIMULATIONS

Games and simulations overlap to some extent with case histories (section 14.9) and also with role playing (section 14.12). So some people may worry about how to define these different teaching methods and worry about deciding whether a particular session is an example of a simulation or a role play or a case history. In fact these worries should not become important. What is important is whether a particular session helps students to learn, not whether it is called a game or a simulation.

The essence of a simulation exercise is that the real world is simplified or reproduced in the classroom. So when students practise injections by injecting an orange, the orange simulates the real skin and muscle of a human being. Simulations can be in a printed form, or, increasingly nowadays, on a computer. In the use of simulations in teaching, the student does something to the simulator and the simulator will respond in some way rather like the real world.

This is a rather complicated attempt to describe in general terms what a simulation is. Examples probably make the idea more easy to understand. In one simulation exercise, the students are put in charge of an imaginary undeveloped country. The country is so undeveloped that at the moment there are no hospitals or health centres. The students are given a budget and told the costs of employing Community Health Workers, or running health centres and hospitals. They are asked to decide how many hospitals they will build, how many health workers they will employ and where they will all be placed in the country.

They are then given cards which each represent one patient and told what disease the patient has, what level of treatment is needed and where the patient lives. The students can then find out how well their health system works with the simulated patients.

The value of the game is that it helps students to think about how to make decisions concerning the allocation of health resources. It also provides some feedback about what happens with different types of health system. (In this simulation, students who spend too much money on regional hospitals find that the coverage of rural areas is poor and so many people die.)

This simulation is used by the authors and has been based on an article published in *Medical Teacher*, Vol. 2 No. 1 in 1980 which was written by H. R. Folmer.

Games are often also simulations. They have the added characteristic that there is some kind of scoring or competition between players. So in a 'Village Health Centre' Game developed at the BLAT Centre in London, the players are in charge of a village health centre. Each player has a counter which moves round a board (as in Monopoly). When the counter lands on a square, the player is given choices about how to spend his time (studying about health care, conducting immunisation programmes, seeing patients, etc.). On other squares things happen, such as an outbreak of measles in a neighbouring village. In this case the player will receive a penalty unless he has previously spent time on a measles immunisation campaign. The players can also pick up 'patient cards' which give the signs and symptoms of the patient. If the player makes a correct diagnosis, then he is considered to have successfully treated that patient. The winner is the player who successfully treats most patients.

This combines practice in reaching decisions about diagnosis with practice in decision making about how to spend time in a health centre. It shows how it is necessary to spend some time in preventive health care and in continuing education even when there are a lot of patients in need of curative treatment.

Another type of game is the 'Clinic Game'. This is best linked to the use of flowcharts. One student is given a card with a list of his signs and symptoms. Another student then asks questions as if he were a health worker in a clinic. He might ask, 'Why have you come to see me?'. The patient might answer 'I'm feeling very tired all day'. The 'health worker' then finds the appropriate flowchart and then asks questions according to the sequence on the flowchart.

This 'Clinic Game' is a good way of teaching students how to make diagnostic or treatment decisions with the help of flowcharts.

14.12 ROLE-PLAY EXERCISES

Role-play exercises have been described in some detail in section 11.10. There they were discussed as a method of teaching attitudes.

Role plays are also very helpful in developing decision-making skills. Obviously whilst any communication is taking place a health worker is continuously making decisions about how much the other person has understood, what would be a good way of explaining the next point, what questions should I ask, etc., etc. These decisions in a role play have to be made at speed and have to be implemented straight away. Thus role play provides excellent practice in making decisions.

14.13 OBSERVED FIELD WORK

Whilst all of the above techniques are useful in developing decision-making skills, they are not enough. A student who has shown ability to make decisions quickly and accurately in all of the *artificial* situations still has not had practice in making decisions in the *real* world. Therefore this sort of practice must be provided.

The principle of providing observed field work is easy. All that is needed is to have the student doing the normal work of a health worker under close supervision. The supervisor is there to protect the community or the individual patient by making sure that the decisions made are correct. The supervisor is also there to provide feedback to the student about whether decisions are correct and to help the student develop more effective methods of reaching decisions. (This means basically pointing out what information or rules have not been taken into account—or pointing out where the thinking has been illogical.)

The supervisor is not there to make the decisions first, nor to collect the information. It must be the student who takes the history or conducts the interview and who first proposes the diagnosis, treatment or course of action.

In order to do this as effectively as possible there should ideally be one supervisor for each student.

All of the above is fairly clear and straightforward. The difficulty is to overcome the enormous practical and financial obstacles in obtaining anything approaching one competent supervisor per student. Suggestions for overcoming this extremely difficult situation are offered in sections 13.5 and 13.6.

14.14 FIELD WORK WITH A SUPERVISOR

The final stage of the practice of decision-making skills is supervised field work. In this situation the student practises the skills without being closely observed. A supervisor is available for the student to refer to in cases of difficulty. The supervisor will also check the work is done by the student and will normally be responsible for the work done by the student.

This kind of situation is normally achieved during substantial periods of attachment in the field. It should perhaps be stressed that the quality of the supervisor is extremely important. It seems reasonable that training institutions should make a major effort to involve service personnel very fully in planning what students should learn during their field attachments. The training institution should also provide training for supervisors so that they can develop their educational skills and can agree on the way in which health care should be provided.

14.15 ASSESSING DECISION-MAKING SKILLS

The principles involved in assessing decision-making skills are again fairly simple. Putting the principles into practice is much more difficult.

The principles are those described in chapter 8. The first principle is that the assessment should test those skills which are used in providing health care (valid assessment). Thus 'Write short notes on how decisions are made in diagnosis' would be totally invalid—even though it seems to have some slight connection with decision making.

Valid assessment can be achieved by using any of the teaching methods as an assessment method. For example, case histories or patient management problems are suitable methods. The only change from the teaching situation is that the student's performance in answering the questions must be recorded and graded by an examiner. Similarly supervised field work can also be used for assessment purposes. The only adaptation needed is for the supervisors to record the grade awarded for each student.

The second principle is that the assessment should be reliable. That is, the grade awarded to a student should fairly reflect that student's ability. Reliability is difficult to achieve, but can be improved by using agreed checklists to observe the student's performance or to mark a student's written work. Another way of increasing reliability is to make a large number of separate assessments. In this way, the inevitable 'errors' which occur in each assessment will tend to cancel out over the series of assessments.

Thus it is suggested that assessment of decision-making skills should be carried out by asking students to perform decision-making tasks which are related to the work of a health worker, this should be done fairly frequently during the course and the scoring of the performance should be guided by a checklist.

One way of organising such an assessment is to use an Objective Structured Practical Examination. This technique is described in detail in chapter 8. Many of the examples given in chapter 8 are either of decision-making skills or can be adapted to test decision-making abilities.

SUMMARY

- Decision making is at the heart of all effective health care.
- Decision-making skills should be taught.
- The sequence for teachers to follow is:
    (i)   analyse the decision-making skills;
    (ii) describe and demonstrate the skills;
    (iii) provide practice in decision making for every learner;
    (iv) assess whether students have learnt.
- Practice in decision making can be provided by using:
    (i)   brain-storming;
    (ii) snowballing;
    (iii) case histories, case studies or patient-management problems;
    (iv) flowcharts;
    (v)   games and simulations;
    (vi) role play;
    (vii) field work.
- Assessing decision-making skills can be done by adapting any of the teaching methods. Reliability is improved if checklists are used to guide the scoring and if assessment is made fairly frequently. The OSPE is one appropriate method for assessing decision-making skills.

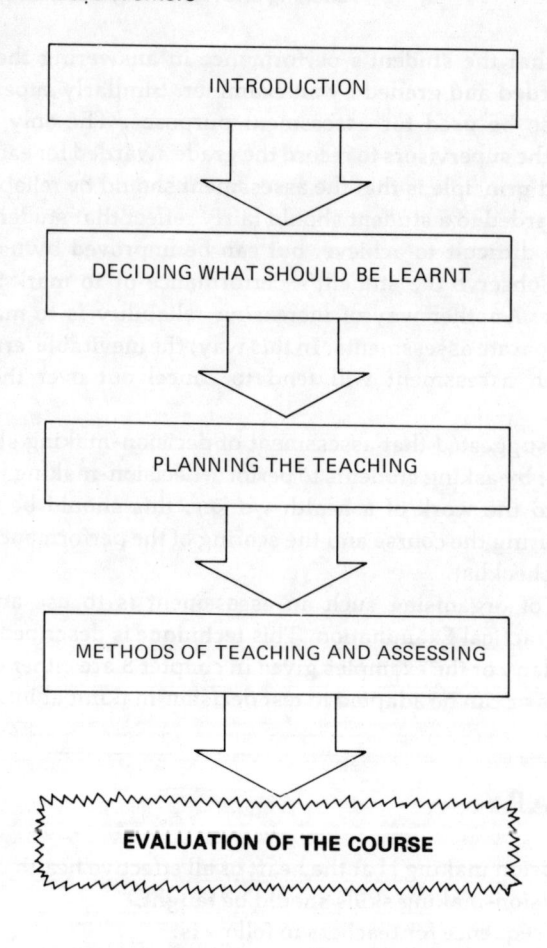

```
     INTRODUCTION
          ↓
DECIDING WHAT SHOULD BE LEARNT
          ↓
   PLANNING THE TEACHING
          ↓
METHODS OF TEACHING AND ASSESSING
          ↓
   EVALUATION OF THE COURSE
```

CONTENTS

15.1	What is the Teacher's Role in Evaluation?	218
15.2	What can be Evaluated?	219
15.3	How to Evaluate the Plan	219
15.4	How to Evaluate the Process	221
15.5	How to Evaluate the Product	228

15
Evaluation of the Course

Evaluation is the process of collecting data about courses and teaching. It is also the process of using this data to reach decisions about ways in which the course should be kept the same or should be changed. So evaluation is different from assessment—which is related to collecting data and making judgements about the individual students.

Evaluation and assessment overlap sometimes. For example, when you carry out a test to find out how much has been learnt at the end of a series of teaching sessions, some of the information is about the performance of individual students and guides their individual learning (e.g. 'Student A scored 65% and needs to learn more about the maintenance of water pumps, but seems competent to build pit latrines'). This is assessment. On the other hand, this same test can tell the teacher that overall the students' average score was 83% and the major weakness was that they did not know how to build protection round a water pump in a village. The teacher now knows that most of the teaching has been quite successful but the section on protection of water supplies should be taught again for this year's students and next year a different approach might be needed. This is evaluation.

Since evaluation is concerned with guiding teaching, it should take place throughout a course and the planning of the course. If evaluation only takes place at the end of a course, it cannot influence that course. This is shown in figure 15.1.

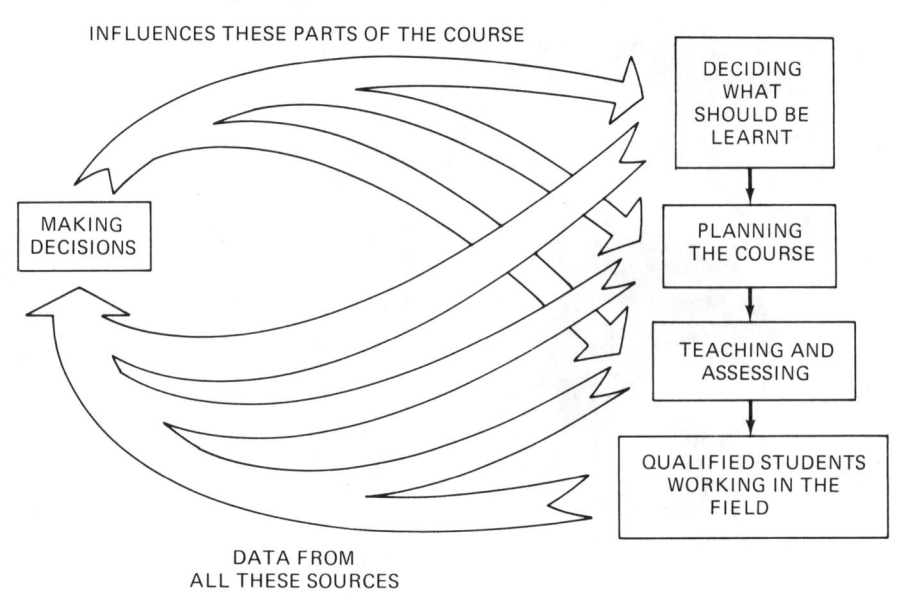

Figure 15.1 The Process of Evaluation. Evaluation takes data from all these sources throughout a course. These data are then used to influence what happens in the course

15.1 WHAT IS THE TEACHER'S ROLE IN EVALUATION?

This chapter is only concerned with what a teacher can do to evaluate the course on which he teaches. The chapter does not attempt to discuss in general how courses can be evaluated, or how an evaluator from outside the course might work.

Rather like assessment, evaluation should be continuous. All the time a teacher should be observing the course and thinking about whether it is going as well as possible. In this way evaluation is a state of mind, rather than a set of techniques.

This questioning and observing approach should be matched with a willingness to accept that teaching can always be done better. Further, the teacher should also be willing to make the effort to improve. With these vitally important attitudes, a teacher will be evaluating himself continually and will probably continue to improve the quality of his teaching throughout his career. Without this willingness to learn and openness to criticism a teacher is most unlikely to improve.

This 'state of mind' continuous evaluation should be supported by some specific activities and can be stimulated by asking particular questions. These activities and questions are described below in sections 15.2–15.5.

Should teachers collect data about all aspects of the course? There seems to be little point in collecting any evaluation data, unless that data could lead to a decision or a change. For example, there is no value in

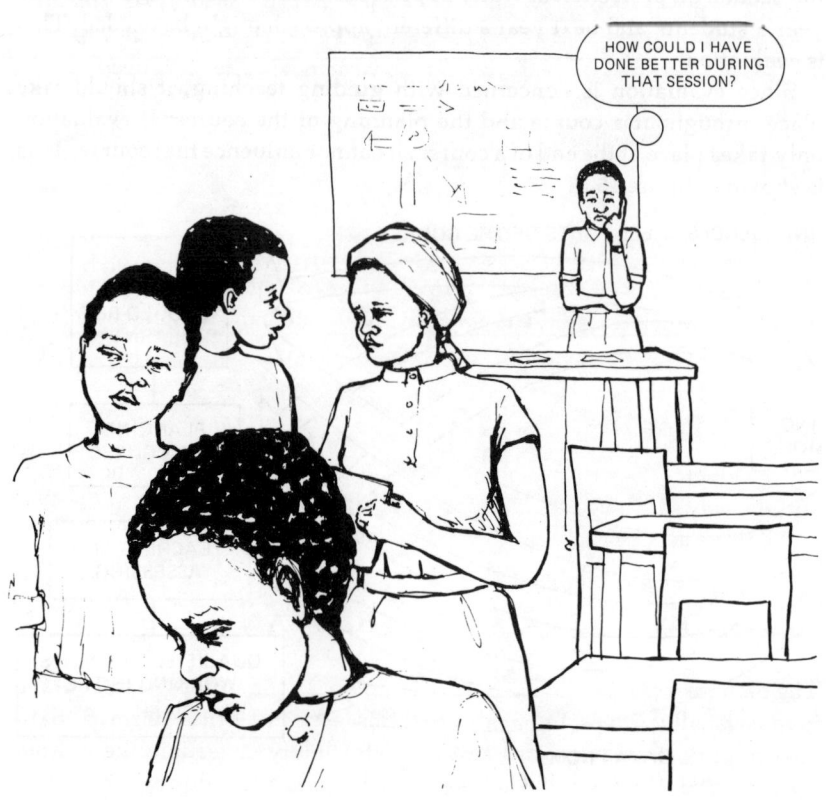

Figure 15.2 Evaluation is a State of Mind

collecting data which show that more detail should be taught in each of the parts of a course, if the length of the course cannot be increased to make time for this more detailed teaching. Similarly there is no point in finding out that 20 new microscopes are needed, unless there is at least some chance that these microscopes could be obtained.

Therefore teachers should direct evaluation efforts at those things which could in principle be changed.

A final point. Evaluation need not point to a need for change. Evaluation can be very useful when it shows current methods are effective and so confirms that theh should continue. This has the benefit of increasing teachers' and students' confidence in what is being done at the moment and allows effort to be concentrated on those places where development is needed.

15.2 WHAT CAN BE EVALUATED

There are three aspects of a course which teachers should evaluate. These are as follows.

(1) The Plan

The plan of the course consists of the overall aim of the course, the stated selection method for choosing students, the learning objectives, the course timetable and the teaching methods which are planned to help students achieve these objectives. Finally there is the assessment plan which is designed to test whether the students have achieved the objectives.

In short, the plan is all those things which can be decided before the course begins and which may—or possibly should—be written down as a plan for the course.

(2) The Process

The process is the way in which the plan is implemented. So this includes the way in which the students actually are selected, the sessions which are taught and the way in which they are taught.

(3) The Product

The product is the outcome of the course. That is, the students who qualify and the way in which they perform as health workers.

All these aspects should be evaluated as far as possible.

15.3 HOW TO EVALUATE THE PLAN

The plan for a course should be written down. In some cases it isn't but the plan is usually well established even if this is not in a written form. So data collection is straightforward and consists simply of reading the written documents or finding out what is planned to take place during a course.

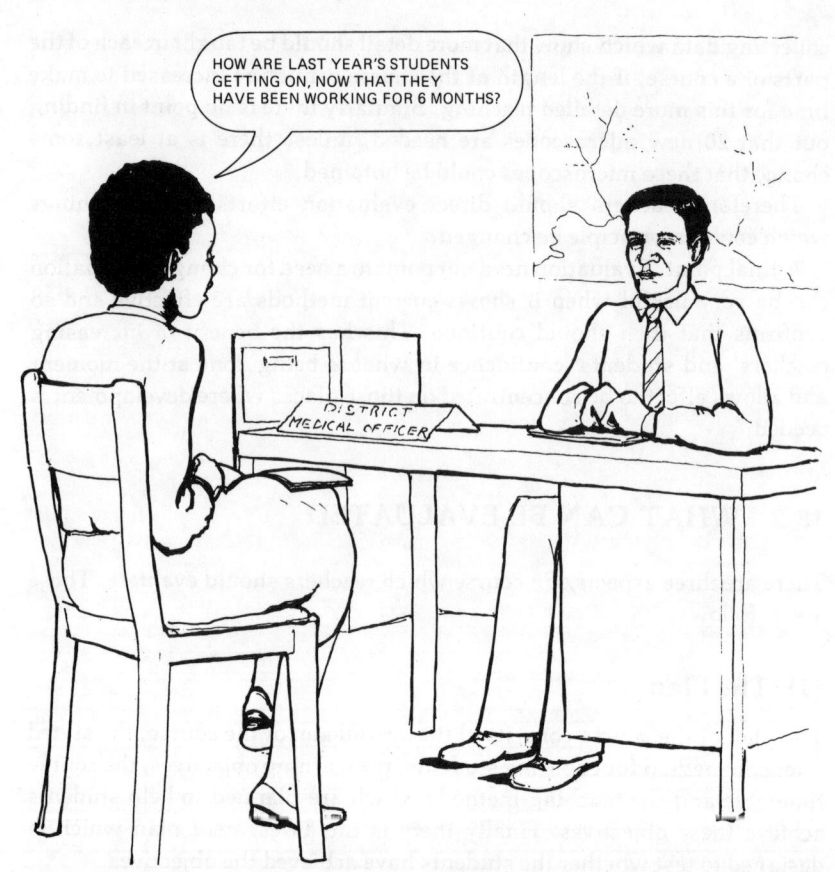

Figure 15.3 Evaluation involves talking to the supervisors of health workers

HOW ARE LAST YEAR'S STUDENTS GETTING ON, NOW THAT THEY HAVE BEEN WORKING FOR 6 MONTHS?

The second stage of evaluation—reaching decisions on the basis of the data collected—is best done in discussion with other teachers. This may be in formal committees or it may be in casual conversation. This decision may be helped by asking some of the following questions.

- Are the students likely to be appropriate? Do they have the right qualifications? Will they be acceptable to the communities where they will work? Will there be the right number? Will they be the right age? Are they likely to be committed to Primary Health Care (PHC)?
- Are the learning objectives appropriate? Are the objectives stated? Do they specify the skills, knowledge and attitudes in sufficient detail? Are the skills, etc., those which are most important in this community? Do the skills, etc., reflect the PHC approach? Can the objectives be learnt within the total time available?
- Does the timetable give a framework in which the learning objectives can be achieved? Is the balance of time between the different parts of the course suitable? Is there enough time allocated to learning communication and decision-making skills? Is there enough time for students to practise skills in the work setting?
- Do the teaching methods chosen seem appropriate for the learning objectives? Is there variety in teaching methods? Are lectures limited to a small proportion of the course? Will the teachers be capable of using the teaching methods specified? Are there suffi-

cient resources (space, equipment, materials, health workers, patients, etc.) to make the methods feasible?
- Will the assessment methods actually test the specified objectives? Are the assessments likely to be valid? Are the assessments likely to be reliable? Will the assessments help the students to learn? Will the assessments concentrate on the most important skills and knowledge? Will the assessments occupy only a small proportion of time? Will the assessments be cheap and feasible?

By asking these questions, other questions are likely to come to mind and the whole plan for the course—or the part of the course for which the teacher is responsible—can be reviewed. These questions are designed to stimulate thought about the course and to focus attention on some of the key issues.

Having considered these questions, the teachers may produce a number of recommendations. These must of course be feasible within resources which are available and should form the first stage in implementing a change in the plan which in turn will lead to changes in the course itself.

15.4 HOW TO EVALUATE THE PROCESS

Ideally, the course should be a direct implementation of the plan. In practice this may not happen for all sorts of reasons. So it is important to collect data about what actually does happen during a course, since this may be rather different to the plan.

The essence of evaluating the plan is to think of the right questions to ask, since the data are usually readily available. When evaluating the process, most of the same questions are appropriate, but the problem is to collect enough and accurate data.

The selection process can be evaluated by studying the students who are selected—and possibly comparing them with the students who are not admitted. The basic question to ask is whether the selection process has achieved the criteria set out in the plan. Often teachers will emphasise intellectual characteristics of students. They will tend to be satisfied if the students are intelligent and have a reasonable background of knowledge. However, these should not be the only criteria for trainee workers in PHC: acceptability within a community, attitudes of service and willingness to share knowledge may be even more important. Data about the students who are selected will only emerge during the course as teachers begin to know the students better. No formal method of data collection (such as interviews or questionnaires) is suggested.

The main area for evaluation is the teaching itself. The underlying questions for this part of the evaluation are:

- Are the times allowed for each part of the curriculum sufficient?
- Is the use of this amount of time as effective as possible (i.e. are the teaching methods appropriate)?
- Is the teaching leading towards the right objectives (i.e. is the content of the teaching session on the right skills and knowledge—is the level of detail appropriate)?

These three aspects, which are clearly quite distinct in principle, tend to become confused in the students' view of a course and often confused by evaluators. For example, a part of the course taught with great enthusiasm and using active learning methods will often be thought of as also covering important objectives at the right level of detail—even when this is not the case. Therefore collecting data about the process of the course must attempt to distinguish between these three aspects.

Data can be collected by:

- observation by the teacher himself;
- observation by other teachers;
- questionnaires completed by students;
- evaluation discussions with students;
- staff meetings.

Examples of these methods are given below.

Observation by the Teachers

As mentioned above, teachers should continuously observe their own performance. This observation can be helped by a checklist for the teacher to fill in at the end of a session or the end of a course. This same checklist can also be filled in by a colleague who sits in on the session. This checklist can then provide a basis for discussion about how future sessions can be improved.

An example of a checklist is given in table 15.1 which can be adapted to suit specific teaching situations. Broadly the more 'yes' responses the better. It should be noted that it is very unlikely that 'yes' can be achieved for every question in any one teaching session. Another point is that often the accurate answer to a question will be 'Yes, but not as often or as well as might have been achieved'. So the checklist is a guide to stimulate teachers to think about how they can improve. A 'yes' response is not necessarily good enough.

Another source of data in evaluation is to observe the students during a teaching session. This can again be helped by using a checklist and this can be filled in either by the teacher himself or by a colleague. After the teaching session the results can be discussed to analyse the reasons. What went well? Why did things go wrong? A guide which may help teachers to observe the students is given in table 15.2.

Questionnaires Completed by Students

It is often difficult for teachers to invite students to comment on the teacher's skill as a teacher. After all, the teacher is a professional and in comparison the students may know much less about teaching. However, students can and do provide very useful guidance when they are given the right atmosphere and some guidance on what to look for. The students do provide a different point of view and ultimately what the student learns is the only criterion for deciding whether teaching is effective.

Table 15.1   Teaching/learning checklist

Clarity of Presentation

	Yes	No
Were the objectives clearly stated?	☐	☐
Were all visual materials clear?	☐	☐
Was the teacher audible?	☐	☐
Were the words used easily understood?	☐	☐
Were important points emphasised and minor details left out?	☐	☐
Was the structure and sequence clear and appropriate?	☐	☐

Making the Learning Meaningful

	Yes	No
Were the objectives worthwhile and appropriate?	☐	☐
Did the teacher find out how much was already known?	☐	☐
Was the learning related to the learners' previous experience?	☐	☐
Was the learning related to the learners' future life?	☐	☐
Were many examples given?	☐	☐
Were underlying principles provided?	☐	☐

Making the Learning Active

	Yes	No
Were all students actively involved in discussion, answering questions, solving problems or practising skills?	☐	☐
Were the teachers' questions designed to provoke thought?	☐	☐
Were standards of performance set or agreed?	☐	☐

Providing Feedback

	Yes	No
Were students given individual advice about how to improve their performance?	☐	☐
Was the feedback immediate?	☐	☐

Checking for Mastery

	Yes	No
Did the teacher check whether learners have achieved the objective?	☐	☐

The Overall Approach of the Teacher

	Yes	No
Did the teacher convey enthusiasm and interest in the subject?	☐	☐
Did the teacher demonstrate interest in the students as people?	☐	☐
Did the teacher have a suitable manner and way of speaking?	☐	☐
Was the relationship between teacher and learner relaxed and non-authoritarian?	☐	☐

Adapted from
Teaching for Better Learning, F.R. Abbatt, WHO, Geneva, 1980.

Table 15.2 *Focus on student behaviour*

Please indicate the proportion of students who fit each of the categories below and add comments in the space provided.
1. *Understanding the aim of the session*   Understand ☐ Puzzled ☐ Indifferent ☐
2. *Enthusiasm to participate in the learning activities*   Motivated ☐ Bored ☐ Indifferent ☐
3. *Attention in class*   Attentive ☐ Not attentive ☐ Not observable ☐
4. *Satisfaction with answers to the question*   Satisfied ☐ Not satisfied ☐ Not applicable ☐
5. *Reaction to other students' contributions to discussion*   Welcome ☐ Bored ☐ Indifferent ☐
6. *Freedom to ask questions*   Felt free ☐ Discouraged ☐ Not observable ☐
Other comments:

Adapted from *Self-assessment for Teachers of Health workers: How to be a Better Teacher*, Arie Rotem and Fred Abbatt, WHO, Geneva, 1982.

Students can be helped in commenting by giving them a questionnaire. An example is given in table 15.3—which again should be used to stimulate the teacher to improve his performance. The questionnaire could be used after just one session, but might be more useful after a series of teaching sessions on one subject.

The questionnaire shown is fairly detailed. It could be usefully simplified in some situations. In any situation teachers should adapt questionnaires to suit their needs.

Evaluation Discussions with Students

It is often useful to discuss courses with students. Questionnaires can give the answers to the teacher's questions; discussions give students more opportunity to discuss the questions which they feel are important.

Table 15.3 *Teaching skills questionnaire*

	Very skilfully	Satisfactorily	Poorly	Not observed in this course	Comments
Please Tick the Appropriate Space During the session/course the teacher was able to:					
1. Explain clearly	☐	☐	☐	☐	
2. Simplify complex issues	☐	☐	☐	☐	
3. Distinguish between important and unimportant issues	☐	☐	☐	☐	
4. Adapt teaching and language to level of students' ability	☐	☐	☐	☐	
5. Summarise issues before moving on	☐	☐	☐	☐	
7. Ask students to apply the knowledge to realistic problems	☐	☐	☐	☐	
8. Pose thought-provoking questions	☐	☐	☐	☐	
9. Arouse interest/curiosity	☐	☐	☐	☐	
10. Inspire and motivate	☐	☐	☐	☐	
11. Encourage participation	☐	☐	☐	☐	
12. Encourage students to share ideas and experiences	☐	☐	☐	☐	
13. Relate issues to the real world	☐	☐	☐	☐	
14. Provide stimulating materials	☐	☐	☐	☐	
15. Provide relevant materials	☐	☐	☐	☐	
16. Detect confusion and misconception	☐	☐	☐	☐	
17. Detect when students are bored	☐	☐	☐	☐	
18. Listen to students sympathetically	☐	☐	☐	☐	

19. Overall did you feel that you learnt:
    a lot (i.e. more than average for a session of this length) ☐   about average ☐   less than average (for a session of this length) ☐

20. Overall was the session:
    taught very well ☐   about average ☐   taught poorly ☐

Adapted from *Self-assessment for Teachers of Health Workers: How to be a Better Teacher*, Arie Rotem and Fred Abbatt, WHO, Geneva, 1982.

Such discussions can be unstructured and totally informal. These discussions can be very helpful to teachers wherever the discussion takes place in an atmosphere of trust and confidence. But even in these circumstances, there is the danger that the students who are most willing to talk are likely to be untypical of the students as a whole. So in addition to informal discussions a structured evaluation discussion is suggested.

This can best be done in the stages described in table 15.4.

Table 15.4 A structured evaluation discussion

Stage 1

Describe to the students the procedure outlined below.

Stage 2

Ask each student to write down a few statements about the course. They should be encouraged to write down the things which they feel are most important. The statements should be fairly specific. For example, the statement 'the course was good' is not nearly specific enough. The way in which it was good should be expressed, so for example a more useful statement might be 'the course objectives were appropriate to my needs'.
It does not matter whether the statement is thought to be true—or the opposite of the truth—since this is dealt with in Stage 4. This means that an equally suitable form of the statement above would be 'the course objectives were *not* appropriate to my needs'. (This partially overcomes the natural reluctance of students to make critical comments.)

Stage 3

Record the statements prepared by each of the students on an OHP transparency or a chart.
At this stage they should be discussed with regard to whether their meaning is clear, but *not* with regard to whether they are true.
Always there will be a lots of overlap between statements from different members of the group, so a lot of statements can be left out without losing important ideas.
The statements should be written so that there is space for five columns to the right of the statements. These columns are used in Stage 4. At the end of Stage 3, you should have a transparency or chart which looks like the following:

Evaluation of the Course 'Health Data'

	Strongly agree	Agree	No opinion	Disagree	Strongly disagree
The day spent in interviewing was very valuable	☐	☐	☐	☐	☐
More time should have been allowed for students to do calculations	☐	☐	☐	☐	☐
The notes on 'Statistical Calculations' were helpful	☐	☐	☐	☐	☐
The reasons for using health data were well explained	☐	☐	☐	☐	☐
The reference textbook is too complicated	☐	☐	☐	☐	☐

Stage 4

In this stage, the students express their own opinion about each statement by voting. When the statements are clearly written and understood the students are asked to decide whether they 'strongly agree', 'agree', 'have no opinion', 'disagree' or 'strongly disagree' with each statement. They vote by showing hands and you must insist that hands are raised high to make your counting easy and quick. To help the voters, you should make sure all have decided on their opinion before you ask for the first group who 'strongly agree' to raise their hands. Then go on to ask who 'agrees' with the statement, and so on. This may sound a little tedious, but about twenty statements can be reviewed in a one-hour session using this technique.

Evaluation of the Course 'Health Data'

	Strongly agree	Agree	No opinion	Disagree	Strongly disagree
The day spent in interviewing was very valuable	9	11	4	5	1
More time should have been allowed for students to do calculations	3	8	12	7	—
The notes on 'Statistical Calculations' were helpful	4	17	2	3	4
The reasons for using health data were well explained	2	10	3	8	7
The reference textbook is too complicated	12	7	6	4	1

Stage 5

The voting can be reviewed and reasons for voting one way or the other may be discussed.

This basic procedure can be adapted by:

(i) inserting the teacher's own statements and so achieving some of the benefits of a questionnaire.
(ii) Arranging for a student to conduct the session and thereby avoid the difficulty of having the teacher influence how students vote. In this case the teacher may come in to discuss the results without knowing which individual students agreed or disagreed with a statement.

This approach is quick, allows students to express ideas on what they feel is important, and is democratic in that each student has an equal say.

Staff Meetings

It is always useful for staff to meet on a regular basis to discuss the progress of the course and identify ways in which the course can be improved. In a three-month course which the authors are involved with, the staff meet for one hour every week to review progress, identify problems and suggest solutions. In addition a long evening meeting takes place at the end of each course to identify ways in which the next course can be made better. All these meetings take into account the evaluation data collected using the kinds of methods described above.

It seems that virtually every course would benefit from having a team of 3–5 teachers who have overall responsibility for the day-to-day running of the course. This team should meet regularly and frequently to review all of the available data about the course and use this data in making decisions about how the course is run.

The essence of evaluating the process of a course is to collect as much data as possible (within the time available) and use these data to make decisions and to implement improvements.

15.5 HOW TO EVALUATE THE PRODUCT

One could argue that if the product is satisfactory, then the process and the plan must also be sufficient. Therefore evaluation of the product is the only important evaluation.

This argument is only partly accurate. It is true that the whole point of organising and teaching a course is to produce effective PHC workers. But it can take several years to find out whether a PHC worker is effective or not. There is also the point that if you find that a PHC worker is not effective, you then need to evaluate the process and the plan to find out what went wrong. So all stages should be evaluated.

Teachers tend to evaluate the 'product' in terms of examination performance at the end of a course. So if the students do well in the examination it is assumed that the course is satisfactory.

It is suggested that teachers extend this evaluation to before the final examination and after it.

The assessment sections of chapters 10–14 give ways of assessing individual student's knowledge, skills and attitudes. The data obtained in this way throughout the course is also available for evaluation purposes. So teachers should use this assessment data to help them evaluate the quality of the teaching and identify aspects which need improving.

After the course, teachers should also meet the PHC workers in the field and talk. Talk about the course and which parts were useful. Talk about what parts of the course have been forgotten—and whether this matters. Talk about the work now being done—and whether the course was a good preparation. Talk about the people who were effective teachers—and what made them good.

The talking should not be restricted to the health workers themselves, but can also include health service managers and supervisors. In this way the link between training and service can be made stronger.

This approach of just talking may seem a little haphazard. It certainly would not be sufficient as the basis for a scientific research paper. But equally a full scale evaluation is not possible; teachers have too many other things to do. So do not be discouraged from using the informal conversation. It will provide some data and some insights. It may stimulate new ideas or questions. It will certainly help teachers to see a little more of how the course relates to work in the field.

SUMMARY

It may seem that a whole range of evaluation techniques have been suggested and that it is impractical to expect teachers to use them. It would be impractical to expect teachers to use all these methods. What is suggested is as follows.

- Teachers should adopt an 'evaluation state of mind', i.e. they should always be observing what is happening and always thinking about how things could be improved.
- Teachers should use at least one or two of the specific techniques mentioned to support the continuous but unstructured observation.
- Teachers should talk about the course:
    with other teachers;
    with students;
    with former students who are now working in the field.

Appendix 1
Resources for Primary Health Care Teachers

A great variety of resources for training PHC workers is available in the world today. But very often the schools and institutes in developing countries do not have the information needed to obtain these resources. This appendix is intended to supply teachers with the addresses of publishers and agencies who produce books, manuals, visual aids (slides and posters), journals and newsletters relevant to PHC training.

A teacher need not be discouraged from applying for resources by lack of finance. Many journals are distributed free of charge and certain agencies give grants for educational materials. WHO and UNICEF have offices and representatives in the capital city of most developing countries and they will assist with certain materials when approached through the Ministry of Health.

1A INTERNATIONAL AGENCIES WHICH SUPPLY PRIMARY HEALTH CARE RESOURCES

Teaching Aids at Low Cost (TALC)
TALC sells teaching aids for health workers at or below cost price. It has a select list of books related to Primary Health Care and sets of slides on a variety of health topics together with explanatory scripts.

The lists of books and slides and instructions on how to order are obtained from:

TALC,
PO Box 49,
St Albans,
Herts AL1 4AX, England

TALC materials are among the best available in the Primary Health Care field and because it is a non-profit organisation they are also among the cheapest.

African Medical and Research Foundation (AMREF)
PO Box 30125,
Nairobi, Kenya

or

London House,
68 Upper Richmond Road,
London SW15 2RP

AMREF produces a series of manuals called *Rural Health Series*.

Appropriate Health Resources and Technologies Action Group (AHRTAG)
    85 Marylebone High Street,
    London W1M 3DE, England

AHRTAG has several publications, and distributes *Diarrhoea Dialogue* free, monthly.

Salubritas
    American Public Health Association,
    International Health Programs,
    1015 15th St. NW,
    Washington DC 10005, USA

Salubritas produces a free Newsletter with information about health programmes throughout the world.

CONTACT
    Christian Medical Commission,
    World Council of Churches,
    150 Route de Ferney,
    1211 Geneva 20, Switzerland

A quarterly journal issued free on request with articles on Primary Health Care experience from various countries.

International Planned Parenthood Federation (IPPF)
    18–20 Lower Regent Street,
    London SW1 4PV, England

Free health education material and pamphlets on family planning.

War on Want
    467 Caledonian Road,
    London N7 9BE

This organisation will fund small-scale development projects overseas, and publishes a few pamphlets on health issues.

Overseas Book Centre
    321 Chapel Street,
    Ottawa, Ontario,
    Canada, K1N 7Z2

Free books available on health topics.

The World Bank
    Health Section,
    1818 H Street NW,
    Washington DC, 20433, USA

Have a list of publications on development and health topics, some of which are free.

The World Health Organization
    1211 Geneva 27,
    Switzerland

Has a wide range of publications related to Health, Primary Health Care, Training and Management. Place requests through the office of WHO in the capital city.

UNICEF

Provides models, slides, posters, first aid kits, projectors and other materials for health training in developing countries.

Applications to UNICEF must be made through the Ministry of Health.

Ross Institute
    London School of Hygiene and Tropical Medicine,
    Keppel/Gower Street,
    London WC1E 7HT

Publishes a series of useful pamphlets on Prevention of Disease, Water Supplies and Sanitation.

1B SELECTED BOOKS AND MANUALS RELATED TO PRIMARY HEALTH CARE

Below are a few books related to Primary Health Care selected by the authors as a guide to teachers who are commencing work in this area. Many more books are available. Lists of books can be obtained from the publishers at the addresses listed.

Title	Author	Publisher
1 Community Health Care in the Developing World		
Medical Care in Developing Countries	M. King	OUP
Health in the Developing World	J. Bryant	Cornell University Press
Health by the People	K. Newell	WHO
Community Diagnosis and Health Action	J. Bennett	Macmillan
An Introduction to the Primary Health Care Approach in Developing Countries	G. Watt & P. Vaughan	Ross Institute
Community Health	C. Wood	AMREF
Community Health Workers Manual	E. Wood	AMREF
2 Health Education		
Applied Communication	A. Fugelsang	Dag Hammarskjold Foundation
Health Education	N. Scotney	AMREF
Visual Communication	D. Saunders	Lutterworth Educational
3 Nutrition		
Human Nutrition in Tropical Africa	Latham	FAO
Nutrition for Developing Countries	King *et al.*	OUP
See How They Grow	D. Morley	Macmillan
Breast Feeding	G. J. Ebrahim	Macmillan

Title	Author	Publisher

4 Immunisation

Pamphlets of the Expanded Immunisation Programme		Available from WHO
How to Look after a Refrigerator		AHRTAG

5 Maternal and Child Health and Family Planning

Midwifery Manual	Fensom	OUP
Obstetric Emergencies	J. Evrett	AMREF
Primary Child Care, Book 1	M. King et al.	OUP
Child Health	Baldin et al.	AMREF
Child Health in the Tropics	Jelliffe	Edward Arnold
Child Care in the Tropics	G. Ebrahim	Macmillan
Paediatric Priorities in the Developing World	D. Morley	Butterworths
Family Planning Pamphlets		IPPF, London

6 Water and Sanitation

Rural Sanitation	Cairncross & Feacham	Ross Institute
Small Water Supplies		
Water Treatment and Sanitation (Simple Methods for Rural Areas)	Mann & Williamson	Intermediate Technology Publications Ltd.
Appropriate Technology for Water Supply and Sanitation	Feacham et al.	World Bank
Sanitation without Water	Winblad & Kilama	Macmillan Education

7 Control of Endemic Disease

Preventive Medicine for the Tropics	Lucas & Gilles	OUP
Tropical Diseases	Wright	E & S Livingstone
Communicable Disease	Eshuis & Manschott	AMREF

8 Diagnosis, Laboratory and Treatment

The Primary Health Care Worker		WHO
Where There is No Doctor	Werner	Macmillan
Diagnostic Pathways	Essex	Churchill Livingstone
Management Schedules for Clinics	Petit	AMREF
Medical Assistants Manual	Wyatt & Wyatt	McGraw-Hill
First Aid	St Johns Ambulance	
A Laboratory Manual for Rural Tropical Hospitals	Cheesbrough	WHO

9 Drugs

Essential Drugs	Technical Report, Series 641	WHO
Therapeutics	Yudkin et al.	Macmillan Education
Drug Dosage for Health Extension Officers		Ministry of Health, Port Moresby, Papua New Guinea

10 Education and Management

Educational Handbook	J. J. Guilbert	WHO
Teaching for Better Learning	F. Abbatt	WHO (available from AMREF)
Helping Health Workers Learn	D. Werner	Macmillan Education
On Being in Charge	McMahon et al.	WHO

Addresses of Publishers

Oxford University Press (OUP).
37 Dover Street,
London W1.
or
Walton Street,
Oxford OX2 6DP.

World Health Organization,
see Appendix 1A.

Macmillans,
Houndmills,
Basingstoke,
Hants RG21 2XS.

Ross Institute,
see Appendix 1A.

AMREF,
see Appendix 1A.

Dag Hammarskjold Foundation,
distributed by:
Almqvist & Wiksell International,
Box 45150 Drottninggatan,
108 S-104 30 Stockholm,
Sweden.

Food and Agricultural Organisation
(FAO),
Via delle Terme di Caracalla,
00100 Rome,
Italy.

Edward Arnold Ltd,
41 Bedford Square,
London WC1B 3DQ.

Butterworth & Co. Ltd,
88 Kingsway,
London WC2B 6AB.

International Planned Parenthood
Federation (IPPF)
see Appendix 1A.

Intermediate Technology
Publications Ltd,
9 King Street,
London WC2E 8HN.

World Bank,
see Appendix 1A.

E. & S. Livingstone,
Robert Stevenson House,
1–3 Baxter's Place,
Leith Walk,
Edinburgh EH1 3AF.

Churchill Livingstone,
Robert Stevenson House,
1–3 Baxter's Place,
Leith Walk,
Edinburgh EH1 3AF.

McGraw-Hill & Co Ltd,
34 Dover Street,
London W1.

AHRTAG,
see Appendix 1A.

Appendix 2
Procedures

NURSING

Take and record temperature.
Take and record pulse rate.
Take and record blood pressure.
Prepare a dressing tray.
Dress a wound.
Remove stitches.
Sterilise syringes and needles.
Give intramuscular injection and/or hypodermic injections.
Change bedlinen.

To be Observed

(These procedures are sometimes observed during the training period to help the auxiliary to understand the things which happen when he refers his patients to hospital. But they are not usually performed in health centres.)
Routine for bedsore prevention.
Bed bath.
Mouth toilet.
Sterilisation of linen gloves and instruments.
Disinfection of rooms.

LABORATORY

Microscopic stool examination.
Venepuncture.
Thick and thin blood slide.
Fields stain.
Giemsa stain.
Haemoglobin estimation.
ESR.
Blood group.
Cross match.
Sickling test.
Collect midstream urine.
Biochemical urine routine.
Microscopic urine.
Urethral smear.
Grams stain.
Collect sputum.
Do leprosy skin smear.
Stain with Ziehl Neelsen.

To be Observed

WBC total and differential.
Examination of the CSF.
Serological tests.

WARD PROCEDURES

Passing a gastric tube.
Intravenous drip.
Other drips.
Catheterisation.
Lumbar puncture.
Paracentesis.
Administering oxygen.

To be Observed

Cut-down (venesection).
Pleural aspiration.
Weight traction.
Gallows traction.
Suprapubic bladder aspiration.

OUTPATIENT AND SURGICAL PROCEDURES

Immunisations
    Smallpox
    BCG
    Triple
    Polio
    Measles.
Child weighing and graphing.
Mid-arm circumference.
Stitch a wound.
Open an abscess.
Extract a tooth.
Instil eyedrops.
Apply an arm sling.
Apply plaster of paris.
Auroscope examination.
Assist at operation.
Intravenous pentothal.

To be Observed

Proctoscopy.
Application of benzyl benzoate.
Dry swabbing of ears.
Reduction of a fracture.
Circumcision.
Tissue biopsy.
Open ether anaesthesia.
EMO machine.
Spinal anaesthesia.
Endotracheal intubation.

Appendix 3
Continuing Education

The emphasis throughout this book has been on the *initial* training of Primary Health Care (PHC) workers. Yet much of what has been said applied equally to the continuing education of these health workers. This Appendix attempts to explain why continuing education is of great importance, how the educational process differs between initial and continuing training, and how PHC teachers can contribute in this important area.

THE IMPORTANCE OF CONTINUING EDUCATION

In recent years there has been a major expansion in the number of health workers trained. Today the number of doctors and nurses who are trained every year is far greater than it was even 10 or 15 years ago. There has also been a major change in that new cadres of health personnel have been introduced and trained in large numbers. Therefore the vast majority of today's health workers have been trained within the past ten years or so. Their knowledge is reasonably up-to-date and their memory of their initial training is fairly clear.

In ten years' time nearly all of this group will still be providing health care. Yet their initial training will be 10 more years out-of-date and their memory of it will be less clear. Unless active measures are taken, the natural trend will be towards a poorer quality of health care. This, therefore, is one fundamental purpose of continuing education—to provide training in the skills of health care so that the quality of health care can be maintained or improved.

Another purpose is to compensate for weaknesses in the initial training. It almost always happens that students master only a proportion of the skills taught during a course. It is also very common for courses to cover only a proportion of the skills needed in the field. Some form of continuing education is needed to correct these weaknesses.

A third purpose is to help the implementation of policy changes in the health care system. Minor changes are often communicated in the form of circulars. More major changes may be described in longer documents. In either case the change will only be implemented if the health worker accepts the change and also has the skill to implement it. Quite often this is not the case. So continuing education is needed to help the implementation of managerial decisions.

A fourth purpose is to prepare health staff for promotion or a change of job.

New techniques or drugs will also imply a need for continuing education.

For all these reasons—and several less important ones—effective continuing education is an essential part of any successful health care system.

WHO SHOULD CARRY OUT A CONTINUING EDUCATION PROGRAMME

An ideal health care system would have a Continuing Education Department which would be responsible for co-ordinating all the continuing education activities. This department would not necessarily do all the teaching, but would

- determine the needs for continuing education in terms of who needed to learn and exactly what they should learn;
- organise educational programmes which would meet these needs;
- evaluate the success of the educational programme.

In most health care systems this department does not exist, or is only partially effective. Therefore all PHC teachers should think about whether they ought to be involved with service personnel in organising continuing education.

In all cases, the PHC teachers are likely to be involved in providing some of the educational activities of the health care system. So it is important to understand some of the problems in providing continuing education and how they can be overcome.

SOME PROBLEMS IN PROVIDING CONTINUING EDUCATION

Continuing education is different from initial training in several respects.

(1) The learners are geographically scattered, therefore they must either be brought together to learn (which is inevitably expensive and requires organisation) or the learning experiences must be delivered to the learner. This may be in the form of supervision or 'distance learning'. Distance learning techniques include the use of radio and television, manuals, journals or specifically designed teaching programmes sent through the post.

(2) The learners inevitably and rightly have many other responsibilities and activities, therefore the continuing education must win the attention and commitment of the learner. This means that the continuing education must be in as attractive a form as possible and must be seen by the learners to solve problems or meet needs which they are already aware of.

(3) The learners have already been trained and they have field experience. This means that they are likely to be sensitive to any implication in the continuing education that they are not competent. They are likely to identify practical difficulties in implementing new ideas. These factors make the job of the teacher more difficult, but they are really

factors to be welcomed. Teachers should use the pride and experience of the learners by employing more 'participatory methods' in the teaching. This means that the learners should participate by sharing their experience, discussing issues, identifying specific difficulties and, most importantly, suggesting their own solutions.

THE BENEFITS OF CONTINUING EDUCATION

The aims of continuing education programmes should always be to bring about improvements in the way health care is provided in the community.

A weakness of many programmes is that courses or other educational programmes are provided which may lead to an increased theoretical knowledge, but this knowledge is not applied in the day-to-day work of the health worker. Therefore the impact of a continuing education activity should be evaluated.

The evaluation can often be best carried out by asking the learners to report what changes they have made. This is not a very accurate way of finding out what changes occur as the learners may exaggerate what they are doing. On the other hand, asking the learners to evaluate change will stimulate that change.

Another method which should often be adopted in continuing education is to ask at the end of the course or programme what changes the learners think they will be able to implement. This will create some commitment to at least attempt the change—even if it is later rejected.

SUMMARY

Teachers of PHC workers are likely to be involved in some form of continuing education.

In continuing education it is especially important to:

- Concentrate the teaching on solving problems which the learners have identified or recognised.
- Use 'participatory' teaching methods.
- Involve the learners in evaluating what changes occur as a result of the teaching.

Appendix 4
An Example of an Assessment Scheme

The following example is intended to show how the general principles of assessment can be applied in a specific situation.

The situation chosen is a course for Village Health Workers (VHW). This course is attended by about 20 trainees who have primary schooling and have been chosen by their villages. The training consists of 3 separate months based at a health centre with two periods of 1 month working with an experienced health worker in between.

Month 1	Month 2	Month 3	Month 4	Month 5
Health Centre	Field Work	Health Centre	Field Work	Health Centre

The assessment takes a variety of forms, some with the emphasis on helping learning, some with the emphasis on finding out whether the trainee VHW should qualify.

A. CONTINUOUS ASSESSMENT

Throughout all teaching sessions a teaching style is used that requires the trainees to think and to work out reasons and solutions for themselves. The trainees are asked to answer questions, to solve problems, to express their opinions.

Throughout this process the teachers listen to the students' responses, identify what is understood and provide confirmation to the trainees that they are correct. When mistakes occur, the teachers try to analyse what is not understood and attempt to correct this.

This continuous observation, assessment and feedback is used in both the theoretical and the practical/communication parts of the course. It achieves a very active learning environment, guides the students' learning and helps the teacher to make the teaching more purposeful and more suited to the needs of the students.

No records are kept of this informal and continuous assessment. However, the teachers do identify which students learn quickly and which have more difficulty. The students who learn more slowly are given additional help and those who have too much difficulty in learning can be advised that their rate of progress is too slow. (In some situations this may lead on to the advice that the student should not continue with the course.)

B. FIELD WORK ASSESSMENT

During the two months of field work, the trainee VHW works with an experienced health worker called a 'supervisor'. The aim is for each trainee to practise in the field the specific skills learnt at the health centre. So for each of the two months there is a list of tasks which each trainee should practise and which the 'supervisor' should observe and assess.

For each of these tasks there is a checklist which provides a guide to how the task should be carried out. This set of checklists is given both to the supervisor and the trainee.

During the field work period the trainee and supervisor jointly carry out the supervisor's normal work with the trainee doing all the tasks which he/she has been taught at the health centre. During the early part of the field work, the supervisor observes the trainee and gives advice (based on the type of checklist described in section 13.6) about how to improve. Towards the end of the month's field work, performance is assessed more formally and the supervisor fills in a checklist for each of the tasks whilst observing the health worker perform the task in the field situation. These completed checklists are discussed with the trainee. They also form the basis for deciding whether the trainee is competent in decision making, communication and manual skills.

This form of assessment is designed to make the general experience of working in the field into a very purposeful learning experience. The trainee is not just an extra pair of hands who can do the boring jobs and so allow the supervisor to do a little less work; instead the trainee undertakes a whole range of specified tasks and is given regular feedback to improve skills.

This assessment depends on the full co-operation of the supervisor and on the supervisor being skilled in making judgements about the trainee's performance and in explaining in an appropriate way how the trainees can get better. To achieve this the supervisors all take part in a short training programme themselves.

The outcome of this assessment (apart from the improved learning) is a list of the tasks in which each trainee has demonstrated competence in the field.

C. IN-COURSE TESTS

The course includes 3 months spent in training at the health centre. This part of the course is the part where the trainees learn the factual information (knowledge) required for their future job. They also learn the communication skills, decision-making skills and manual skills which they will practise later in the field. All these aspects are assessed.

Every two weeks (i.e. at the middle and at the end of each month) a 1-hour written test is used to assess the knowledge learnt. This consists of short-answer and MCQ items designed to cover the most important facts—not the less important details. The pass mark is 80%. Trainees who do not achieve this mark are allowed to repeat the test at a later date.

The skills (communication, decision-making and manual) are assessed using role-play exercises and patient-management problems which are integrated with the rest of the teaching.

This part of the assessment gives a record of which trainees have passed each of the written tests. The scores and detailed feedback from each assessment is available to each trainee to guide their learning.

D. END-OF-COURSE ASSESSMENT

By the end of the course all trainees who are reasonably well motivated and have the necessary ability will have learnt to be competent in the types of health care for which they are trained. Evidence of this competence is available through the supervisors' reports from the field experience, from the scores on the written in-course tests and from the general impression of teachers during the course.

With all this evidence, end-of-course assessment should be unnecessary as any trainees who are not sufficiently competent will have been identified earlier in the course.

However it often happens that an additional check is needed.

In this situation an oral exam with an assessor who is not one of the course teachers can be used. This assessor should be restricted to asking questions which have appeared on the in-cours tests of knowledge to make sure that the trainee's scores on these tests were a reasonable estimate of the trainee's knowledge. (This restriction prevents the assessor going into too much detail or into areas of knowledge which are not included in the course. Some people might argue that it would be too limited, but as a wide range of the important knowledge has been assessed in these tests, trainees who have mastered these tests will have a good standard of knowledge.)

The skills are assessed in a two hour Objective Structured Practical Exam (OSPE) which assesses each student's ability to carry out parts of 20 different tasks at a series of 'stations'. Their ability is observed at several of these stations using checklists. This OSPE is to confirm that evidence from the field work is accurate.

E. THE OVERALL DECISION

The overall decision to pass or fail the trainees is based on all of these assessments. A trainee should achieve a satisfactory standard in each of the following:

(i) General progress during the course at the health centre.
(ii) Achieving competence in each of the tasks assessed during field work.
(iii) A pass standard on each of the written tests during the course.
(iv) A pass standard in the oral exam.
(v) A pass standard in the OSPE.

Throughout a high pass mark is required (i.e. 80%) with the questions and tests being based on the normal work undertaken by VHWs regularly. The aim is to achieve high competence in the ordinary work of a VHW.

Comment

This may well seem a heavily exam-oriented course. However, in total there are only 6 hours of written tests and 2 hours practical (the OSPE) and an oral assessment in a 5 month course. The remainder of the assessment is based on observing purposefully what the trainee is doing as part of the normal course work or field experience. The strength of this assessment scheme is that the information from all the observation and testing is fed back to the trainees who can then learn more effectively.

Index *

Active learning *112*, 115–118, 132, 222
Adult learning 107
Aims 27
Alma Ata 5, 6
Assessment 20, 24, 74, 80, *Chapter 8*
  choice of method 94
  of attitudes 154–156
  of communication 174–175
  of decision-making skills 214–215
  of knowledge 134–140
  of manual skills 193–195
Attitude scale 155
Attitudes 63–64, *Chapter 11*
Auxiliary health worker 2, 7, 9

Blackboard *see* Chalkboard
Books 126
Brainstorm 116, *205–207*

Case history 209–211
Case study 209–211
Chalkboard 114, *129*
Checklist 63, 92, 95, 164–5, 170, 175, *187–190*, 193, 215, 222
Clinical assistant 2
Communication 10, 18
Communication skills 61, 63, 94, *Chapter 12*
Community 6, 8, 9, 39, 40, 51, 55
  culture *see* Community traditions
  needs 45
  participation 7, 10, 32
  traditions 31, 32
Continuing education 11, 121, Appendix 3
Continuous assessment 83, *89*, 193–195, Appendix 4
Counselling 21
Course programme 74, 112
Criterion-referenced test 88

Critical Incident Study 34
Curriculum 17, 34, 41, 42, 43, 44
Curriculum design 112

Debates 116
Decision making 10
Decision-making skills 10, 63, 68, 94, *Chapter 14*
Demonstrations 115, 119, 164, *181–182*, 203
Diagnostic assessment 89
Diagrams 108
Discussions 107, 148, *166–170*, 207–209, 222

Enabling factors *63–64*, 66, 69
Essays 24, *138*
Evaluation *Chapter 15*
Exams *see* Assessment
Examining Boards 24

Feedback 99, *113*, 135, 155, 172, 174, 183, 185, 187, 192, 223, Appendix 4
Feldsher 2
Field visits 74, *83*
Field work *213*, 214, Appendix 4
Film 114, 149, 158
Flip chart 114
Flowcharts 133, 200, 201, *211*
Freire, Paulo 124

Games 116, *212*

Handouts 82, 112, 115, *131*, 158
Health education 7, 51, *59*
Health for all 5
Health promotion 3

---

* Main entries appear in *italics*.

Index

Immunisation 4, 7, 8, 9, *56,* Appendix 1
Information sources *133,* 134, 140
Intersectoral co-operation 7

Job description *see* Job specification
Job specification 31, 40, 42
Journals 127

Knowledge 61, 63–64, 67, *Chapter 10*

Lesson plan *77*, 112

Manuals 43, 112, 115, 127, 164, 181, 200, Appendix 1
Manual skills 61, 63, 67, 68, 94, *Chapter 13*
Maternal and Child Health 7, 11, 34, 44, 46, 51, *57–58*, 125, Appendix 1
Medical assistant 2
Medical care model 3, 4, 9
Memory game 111
Models 82, 115
Morbidity data 32, 45
Mortality data 32, 45
Motivation 105
Multiple Choice tests 20, 24, 83, 94, 135, *136–138,* Appendix 4

Newsletter 126
Norm-referenced test 89
Nutrition 7, 9, 11, 17, 42, 46, *56–57*

Objective 61, 77, 219, 220
Objective Structured Practical Exam (OSPE) *94–101*, 195, 215, Appendix 4
One-from-five MCQ 137
Open book exam 135, *140*
Oral exam 93, *135*, 174, Appendix 4
Overhead projector 114, 130

Pass mark 93, 134, *194*, Appendix 4
Patient-management problem 139, *209,* Appendix 4
Peer learning 118
Performance skills 63–64
Physical environment for learning 107
Posters 115, 149
Practical session 74, 82–85 *see also* Field Work, Demonstrations and manual skills
Practice exam 93
Practice in pairs 133, 186
Primary Health Care *Chapter 1*, 27, 39, 51–59, 62, 90, 144, 159
Problem solving 53, *54, see also* Decision making
Procedure book 187, 195
Programmed learning 118
Project 83, 118, *173,* 175

Questionnaire 222

Rating scale 95, 135, *154–156,* 172, 175, 187–191, 193–194
Relevance *109, 123*
Reliability *91,* 96, 134, 135, 138, 139, 140, 174, 193, 215
Resources 80, 82, Appendix 1
Role model 150
Role play 117, *151–154,* 170–171, 213, Appendix 4
Roster 186, *192*
Rota *see* Roster

Selection 221
Self-study 118, 130
Short-answer questions 83, 95, *139,* Appendix 4
Simulated patients 99
Simulation 117, 183, *212*
Slides (35 mm) 114, *130*
Snowball discussions 116, *207–209*
Social relationships 107
Sub-task 64–66
Supervision 214
Syllabus 17
Syndicate discussions 116

Tape recording 164
Tape-slide programme 149
Target concept 70, 126
Tasks *Chapter 4, Chapter 5*
Task analysis *Chapter 4, Chapter 6,* 124
Task list 34, 36, *Chapter 4,* 61, 73
Teaching methods
　Active *see* Active learning
　Choice of 119
　for Attitudes Chapter 11
　for Communication skills Chapter 12
　for Decision-making skills Chapter 14

for Knowledge   Chapter 10
for Manual skills   Chapter 13
Testing   *see* Assessment or Evaluation
Time, allocation of   62, 80, 92, 113, 184, 186, 194
Traditional medicine   9
Traditions   *see* Community traditions
True-false type MCQ   137

Validity   *90*, 96, 134, 135, 138, 139, 174, 214
Videotape   164, 173
Visual aids   82, 108, 114, 129

World Health Organization   5
Written exercises   117